ADVANCES IN

Anesthesia

Editor-in-Chief
Thomas M. McLoughlin Jr, MD

ELSEVIER
An Imprint of Elsevier, Inc.
PHILADELPHIA LONDON TORONTO MONTREAL SYDNEY TOKYO

ADVANCES IN
Anesthesia

VOLUMES 1 THROUGH 33 (OUT OF PRINT)

VOLUME 34

VOLUME 35

Preface, *by Thomas M. McLoughlin Jr, Francis V. Salinas, and Laurence C. Torsher*

Postoperative Sleep Disturbances: Understanding and Emerging Therapies, *by David R. Hillman*

Hypothermia: Update on Risks and Therapeutic and Prophylactic Applications, *by Miguel A. Cobas and Arnaldo Vera-Arroyo*

Challenges in the Perioperative Care of Adolescents, *by Lana M. Volz and Bridget L. Muldowney*

Obstetric Hemorrhage: Prevention, Recognition, and Treatment, *by Jason Papazian and Rachel M. Kacmar*

Advances in the Anesthetic Management of Solid Organ Transplantation, *by Christopher L. Wray*

Extracorporeal Membrane Oxygenation, *by Stephen A. Esper*

Quadratus Lumborum Blocks, *by Hesham Elsharkawy*

Complications of Allogeneic Blood Product Administration, with Emphasis on Transfusion-Related Acute Lung Injury and Transfusion-Associated Circulatory Overload, *by Tamara Friedman, Mazyar Javidroozi, Gregg Lobel, and Aryeh Shander*

Practical Management of the Opioid-Tolerant Patient in the Perioperative Surgical Home, *by John-Paul J. Pozek, Stephen F. Goldberg, Jaime L. Baratta, and Eric S. Schwenk*

Practical Management of a Regional Anesthesia-Driven Acute Pain Service, *by Stephen F. Goldberg, John-Paul J. Pozek, Eric S. Schwenk, Jaime L. Baratta, David H. Beausang, and Andrew K. Wong*

Update on Perioperative Pulmonary Embolism Management: A Decision Support Tool to Aid in Diagnosis and Treatment, *by Alan M. Smeltz, Lavinia M. Kolarczyk, and Robert S. Isaak*

VOLUME 36

Preface: Anesthesiology at the Cutting Edge, *by Thomas M. McLoughlin Jr, Laurence C. Torsher, Francis V. Salinas, and Richard P. Dutton*

Care of the Severely Injured Orthopedic Trauma Patient: Considerations for Initial Management, Operative Timing, and Ongoing Resuscitation, *by Justin E. Richards, Bianca M. Conti, and Thomas E. Grissom*

Patient Satisfaction in Anesthesia: Implementation, Relevance, and Identification of Meaningful Measures, *by Anum Wazir, Aesha Shukla, and Richard P. Dutton*

Emergency Preparedness and Mass Casualty Considerations for Anesthesiologists, *by Catherine M. Kuza and Joseph H. McIsaac III*

Optimal Perioperative Blood Pressure Management, *by Senthil Packiasabapathy K and Balachundhar Subramaniam*

Updates in the Management of Postoperative Nausea and Vomiting, *by Anthony L. Kovac*

Left Ventricular Assist Devices and Noncardiac Surgery, *by James A. Nelson, William J. Mauermann, and David W. Barbara*

Neurocognitive Impact of Anesthesia in Children, *by Susan Lei, Riva Ko, and Lena S. Sun*

Update on Modalities and Techniques for Labor Epidural Analgesia and Anesthesia, *by Anthony Chau and Lawrence C. Tsen*

Transversus Abdominis Plane Blocks, *by Nicholas Statzer and Kenneth C. Cummings III*

Cardiac Dysrhythmias: Understanding Mechanisms, Drug Treatments, and Novel Therapies, *by Emily Methangkool, Kimberly Howard-Quijano, and Aman Mahajan*

Perioperative Management of Pulmonary Hypertension and Right Ventricular Failure During Noncardiac Surgery, *by Marco A. Aguirre, Isaac Lynch, and Bailor Hardman*

Trends in Anesthesia-Related Liability and Lessons Learned, *by Juan C. Mora, Alan D. Kaye, Matthew L. Romankowski, Paul J. Delahoussaye, Richard D. Urman, and Rene Przkora*

Director, Continuity Publishing: Taylor E. Ball
Editor: Colleen Dietzler
Developmental Editor: Casey Potter

Printed in the United States of America.

Editorial Office:
Elsevier
1600 John F. Kennedy Blvd,
Suite 1800
Philadelphia, PA 19103-2899

International Standard Serial Number: 0737-6146
International Standard Book Number-13: 978-0-323-69731-6

ADVANCES IN
Anesthesia

MIKE P.W. GROCOTT, BSc, MBBS, MD, FRCA, FRCP, FFICM, Professor of Anaesthesia and Critical Care Medicine, University of Southampton, South Hampton, United Kingdom

CHRISTINE L. HUNT, DO, Assistant Professor of Anesthesiology, College of Medicine, Department of Anesthesiology and Perioperative Medicine, Division of Pain Medicine, Mayo Clinic, Rochester, Minnesota, USA

ROBERT ISAAK, DO, Associate Professor, Assistant Residency Program Director, Department of Anesthesiology, The University of North Carolina at Chapel Hill, Chapel Hill, North Carolina, USA

RAVI JOSHI, MD, FASE, Associate Professor, ACTA Fellowship Program Director, Department of Anesthesiology and Pain Management, The University of Texas Southwestern Medical Center, Dallas, Texas, USA

MELISSA R. KENEVAN, MD, Pain Medicine Fellow, Department of Anesthesiology and Perioperative Medicine, Mayo Clinic, Rochester, Minnesota, USA

KYEONG SEON M. KIM, MD, Assistant Clinical Professor, UC Davis Department of Anesthesiology and Pain Medicine, UC Davis Medical Center, Sacramento, California, USA

A. KENNEDY KOERNER, MAJ, USAF, MD, Physician, U.S. Air Force, Assistant Professor, Department of Anesthesiology, University of Maryland School of Medicine, Center for the Sustainment of Trauma and Readiness Skills (CSTARS)-Baltimore, R Adams Cowley Shock Trauma Center, Baltimore, Maryland, USA

ROBERT SCOTT KRISS, DO, Associate Professor, UC Davis Department of Anesthesiology and Pain Medicine, UC Davis Medical Center, Sacramento, California, USA

JENNY KWAK, MD, Associate Professor, ACTA Fellowship Director, Department of Anesthesiology and Perioperative Medicine, Loyola University Medical Center, Maywood, Illinois, USA

TIM J. LAMER, MD, Professor of Anesthesiology, College of Medicine, Department of Anesthesiology and Perioperative Medicine, Division of Pain Medicine, Mayo Clinic, Rochester, Minnesota, USA

WILLIAM DAVID MAUCK, MD, Assistant Professor of Anesthesiology, College of Medicine, Department of Anesthesiology and Perioperative Medicine, Division of Pain Medicine, Mayo Clinic, Rochester, Minnesota, USA

THOMAS M. McLOUGHLIN Jr, MD, Chair, Department of Anesthesiology, Lehigh Valley Health Network, Allentown, Pennsylvania; Professor of Surgery, Division of Surgical Anesthesiology, University of South Florida Morsani College of Medicine, Tampa, Florida

MICHAEL (MONTY) G. MYTHEN, MD, Smiths Medical Professor of Anaesthesia and Critical Care, University College London, London, United Kingdom

KENNETH E. NELSON, MD, Associate Professor, Department of Anesthesiology, Wake Forest School of Medicine, Winston-Salem, North Carolina, USA

OLUDARE O. OLATOYE, MD, Assistant Professor of Anesthesiology, College of Medicine, Department of Anesthesiology and Perioperative Medicine, Division of Pain Medicine, Mayo Clinic, Rochester, Minnesota, USA

AMIT PAWA, BSc(Hons), MBBS(Hons), FRCA, EDRA, Consultant, Anaesthetic Department, Guy's & St Thomas' NHS Foundation Trust, St Thomas' Hospital, London, United Kingdom

MOHAMED A. REHMAN, MD, Professor of Anesthesiology, Critical Care, and Pediatrics, Chair, Department of Anesthesiology, Johns Hopkins All Children's Hospital, St Petersburg, Florida, USA

JUSTIN E. RICHARDS, MD, Assistant Professor, Department of Anesthesiology, University of Maryland School of Medicine, R Adams Cowley Shock Trauma Center, Baltimore, Maryland, USA

PHILIP E.F. ROMAN, MD, MPH, Department of Anesthesiology, Centura St. Anthony Hospital, United States Anesthesia Partners, Lakewood, Colorado, USA

FRANCIS V. SALINAS, MD, US Anesthesia Partners–Washington; Swedish Medical Center; Clinical Assistant Professor, Department of Anesthesiology and Pain Medicine, University of Washington, Seattle, Washington, USA

RON E. SAMET, MD, Assistant Professor, Department of Anesthesiology, University of Maryland School of Medicine, R Adams Cowley Shock Trauma Center, Baltimore, Maryland, USA

ELIZABETH SCHOLZEN, MD, MHA, Department of Anesthesiology, University of Wisconsin-Madison School of Medicine and Public Health, University of Wisconsin-Madison, Madison, Wisconsin, USA

KRISTOPHER M. SCHROEDER, MD, Associate Professor, Department of Anesthesiology, University of Wisconsin-Madison School of Medicine and Public Health, University of Wisconsin-Madison, Madison, Wisconsin, USA

ALLAN F. SIMPAO, MD, MBI, Assistant Professor, Department of Anesthesiology and Critical Care, University of Pennsylvania Perelman School of Medicine, Children's Hospital of Philadelphia, Philadelphia, Pennsylvania, USA

TIMOTHY J. TAUTZ, MD, Professor, UC Davis Department of Anesthesiology and Pain Medicine, UC Davis Medical Center, Sacramento, California, USA

LAURENCE C. TORSHER, MD, Department of Anesthesiology and Perioperative Medicine, Mayo Clinic, Rochester, Minnesota, USA

NAFISSEH S. WARNER, MD, Assistant Professor of Anesthesiology, College of Medicine, Department of Anesthesiology and Perioperative Medicine, Division of Pain Medicine, Mayo Clinic, Rochester, Minnesota, USA

ANDREW L. WILKEY, MD, Department of Anesthesia, Abbott Northwestern Hospital, Minneapolis, Minnesota, USA

ANGELA M. ZENG, MD, Department of Anesthesiology, University of Wisconsin-Madison School of Medicine and Public Health, University of Wisconsin-Madison, Madison, Wisconsin, USA

DAVID A. ZVARA, MD, Professor, Chair, Department of Anesthesiology, Chief Operating Office, UNC Faculty Physicians, The University of North Carolina at Chapel Hill, Chapel Hill, North Carolina, USA

CONTENTS

VOLUME 37 • 2019

Advances in Anesthesia 37 (2019) xix–xxi

ADVANCES IN ANESTHESIA

ELSEVIER
MOSBY

PREFACE

Anesthesia Practice on the Rise

Check for updates

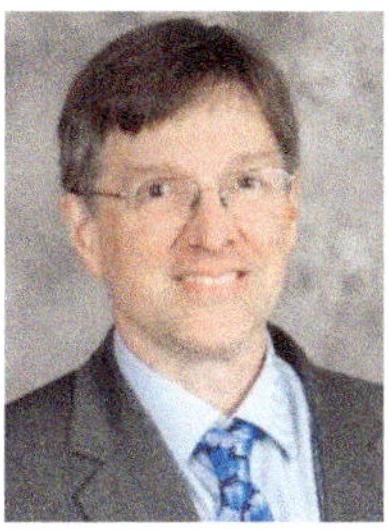
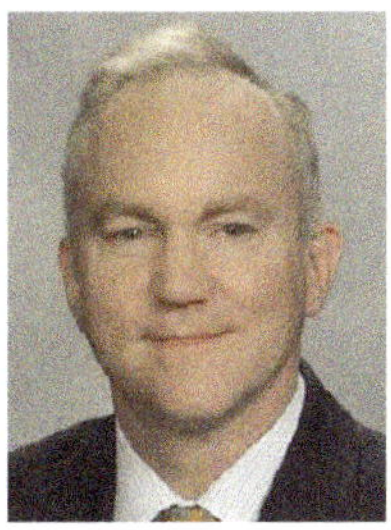
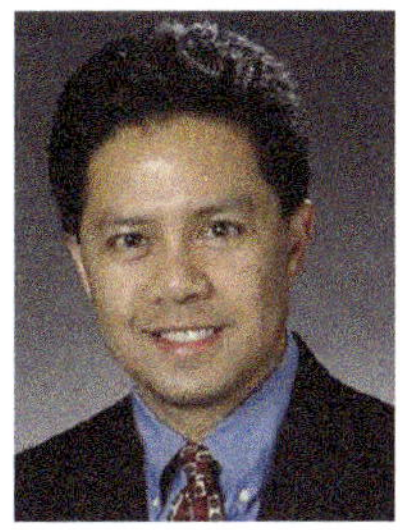
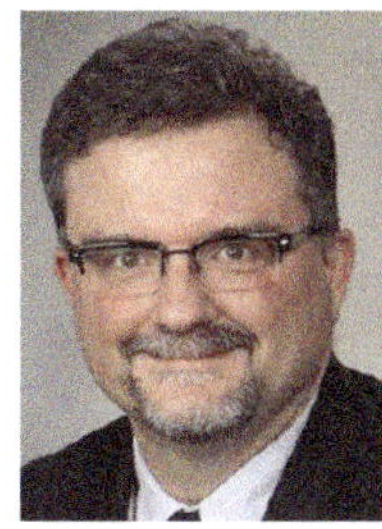

Richard P. Dutton, MD, MBA
Thomas M. McLoughlin Jr, MD
Francis V. Salinas, MD
Laurence C. Torsher, MD
Editors

Welcome to *Advances in Anesthesia*! We are pleased to present you with 11 articles covering topics across the spectrum of perioperative care. These include traditional clinical science articles on management of hemodynamics during cesarean section, treatment of malignant hyperthermia, and perioperative blood conservation; cutting edge information on new regional anesthetic techniques, use of tranexamic acid, and an overview of implanted nerve stimulation technology. In addition, we have included articles that could be drawn directly from our current headlines: diversity in the anesthesia workforce, perioperative management of patients with substance abuse disorder, and a focused look at artificial intelligence and clinical informatics for anesthesiologists.

One unusual article in this year's volume is a Pro:Pro:Pro review of career options for anesthesiologists, team written by 2 academic anesthesiologists, a small-group practitioner, and a representative from the largest private practice in the United States. There is no "con" to this article because overall it's a great time to be an anesthesiologist! Driven by our profession's ability to care for any kind of patient, from neonate (or even in utero) to centenarian, and to facilitate any procedural aspect of modern medicine from electroconvulsive therapy to cardiac transplantation, anesthesiology is at a peak of influence never before achieved. Compensation is good; case numbers are growing, and residency positions are hotly sought after. Any kind of anesthesiology practice today has much to recommend it and represents a smart career choice for the talented

https://doi.org/10.1016/j.aan.2019.09.001
0737-6146/19/© 2019 Published by Elsevier Inc.

medical student. Beyond the overall picture though, we solicited this article to share some hard-won information not commonly found in academic papers or conference presentations. The goal was to compare the benefits and challenges of different anesthesia practice models in a way that will help graduating residents and fellows pick the best spot to launch their own careers, thus helping to keep our profession on the rise.

Longtime readers, and there are many of you, might wonder how topics like this one are chosen. The answer comes directly from our daily experiences in the operating room (OR), intensive care unit, and hospital boardroom. We editors represent clinically diverse practices that span the United States. Dr Torsher is a leader in transplant anesthesia and medical simulation at one of America's most respected academic medical centers as well as a senior editor for the American Society of Anesthesiologist's Self-Education and Evaluation continuing medical education program. Dr Salinas is a clinical leader for a large hospital system in the Pacific Northwest, and the Director of Perioperative Care for the interventional units of his hospital. Dr Dutton is the former Chief Quality Officer of the ASA and currently serves in that role for US Anesthesia Partners. And Dr McLoughlin is a Board Member of the American Board of Anesthesiology and Chief of Anesthesia for an entire hospital system. We are actively engaged with the research, teaching, and pragmatic management of anesthesiology from the level of individual patient care to the management of OR suites to hospital, system, and even national leadership. The articles we solicit each year for *Advances in Anesthesia* address the challenges we are confronting every day in our own work, making it likely they will be relevant to most of our fellow practitioners. But if there's a topic anywhere under the broad roof of perioperative medicine that you'd like to read more about, please don't hesitate to let us know. Our e-mails are published in every issue for a reason!

Finally, thank you for subscribing to this *Advances in Anesthesia*. We appreciate your commitment to remaining current in one of the most dynamic specialties in all of medicine, and we hope you'll find something in this issue to learn from. Whether practical information on a new medication, device, or technique, or thought-provoking discussion of an emerging issue, we've tried to include a wide variety of entertaining and educational content. Enjoy!

Richard P. Dutton, MD, MBA
US Anesthesia Partners
Merit Drive
Dallas, TX 75225, USA

Department of Anesthesiology
Baylor Scott & White Texas A&M College of Medicine
Bryan, TX 77807, USA

E-mail address: Richard.dutton@usap.com

Thomas M. McLoughlin Jr, MD
Department of Anesthesiology
Lehigh Valley Health Network
1200 South Cedar Crest Boulevard
Central Utility Building
Allentown, PA 18103, USA

Division of Surgical Anesthesiology
University of South Florida
Morsani College of Medicine
Tampa, FL 33612, USA

E-mail address: thomas.mcloughlin@lvhn.org

Francis V. Salinas, MD
US Anesthesia Partners–Washington
1229 Madison Street, Suite 1440
Seattle, WA 98104, USA

Swedish Medical Center
Seattle, WA 98122, USA

Department of Anesthesiology and Pain Medicine
University of Washington
Seattle, WA 98195, USA

E-mail address: fvsalinasmd@gmail.com

Laurence C. Torsher, MD
Department of Anesthesiology and Perioperative Medicine
Mayo Clinic Rochester
Rochester, MN 55905, USA

E-mail address: torsher.laurence@mayo.edu

Advances in Anesthesia 37 (2019) 1–34

ADVANCES IN ANESTHESIA

Perioperative Blood Conservation: Guidelines to Practice

Jenny Kwak, MD[a,*], Andrew L. Wilkey, MD[b], Mohamed Abdalla, MD[c], Ravi Joshi, MD[d], Philip E.F. Roman, MD, MPH[e], Philip E. Greilich, MD, MSc[f]

[a]Department of Anesthesiology and Perioperative Medicine, Loyola University Medical Center, 2160 South First Avenue, Maywood, IL 60153, USA; [b]Department of Anesthesia, Abbott Northwestern Hospital, 800 East 28th Street, Minneapolis, MN 55407, USA; [c]Department of Cardiothoracic Anesthesiology, Cleveland Clinic Lerner College of Medicine, Anesthesiology Institute, Cleveland Clinic, 9500 Euclid Avenue/J4-331, Cleveland, OH 44196, USA; [d]Department of Anesthesiology and Pain Management, University of Texas Southwestern Medical Center - Dallas, 5323 Harry Hines Boulevard, Dallas, TX 75390-8894, USA; [e]Department of Anesthesiology, Centura St. Anthony Hospital, United States Anesthesia Partners, 11600 West 2nd Place, Lakewood, CO 80228, USA; [f]Cardiac Anesthesiology, Department of Anesthesiology and Pain Management, University of Texas Southwestern Medical Center - Dallas, 5323 Harry Hines Boulevard, Dallas, TX 75390-8894, USA

Keywords

• Clinical practice guideline • Implementation • Anemia • Transfusion
• Patient blood management • Robust process improvement • Quality improvement
• Survey

Key points

- The formulation of clinical practice guidelines are complex, resource-intense processes for summarizing evidence-based best practices, yet alone are insufficient for translating guidelines to practice.
- The implementation of practice guidelines requires changing physician behaviors, engaging multiple stakeholders with flexible and persistent leadership effort.
- Identifying and responding to both barriers and facilitators of evidence-based best practices are vital to translating guidelines to practice.

Continued

Disclosure Statement: Dr P.E. Greilich has received funding for an investigator-initiated clinical trial from AMAG Pharmaceuticals (United States).

*Corresponding author.

https://doi.org/10.1016/j.aan.2019.08.011
0737-6146/19/

Continued

- Strategies for implementing patient blood management are emerging and represent and opportunity for robust process improvement.
- The coordinated use of a survey instrument for audit and feedback can align local, regional, and national efforts for translation of blood conservation guidelines to clinical practice.

INTRODUCTION

Translating guidelines for perioperative blood conservation and hemostasis to practice is an area of intense interest to anesthesiologists, administrators, patients, and surgeons. In addition to reviewing relevant evidence-based clinical practice guidelines for patient blood management, this article addresses how to overcome barriers and to facilitate the closure of the evidence-to-practice gap. The purpose of this article is to review the data and provide a framework for translating guidelines to practice. The use of a survey instrument to facilitate audit and feedback is highlighted.

FORMULATING CLINICAL PRACTICE GUIDELINES

According to the National Academy of Medicine, clinical practice guidelines are statements that include recommendations intended to optimize patient care and are informed by a systematic review of evidence and an assessment of the benefits and harms of alternative care options [1]. Although the rationale for creating clinical practice guidelines is sound, the formulation of objective, relevant, and easily applied recommendations currently faces many challenges. They are complex, resource-intense undertakings that may overlap with one another and struggle to stay current with new evidence. The number and complexity of guidelines has grown considerably over the past decade. In 2015, the US Agency for Healthcare Research and Quality National Guidelines Clearinghouse listed 2619 individual guidelines on its website [2].

The National Academy of Medicine has a clearly defined and rigorous definition of trustworthy guidelines that distinguishes clinical practice guidelines from other forms of advice such as consensus statements, position papers, practice bulletins, scientific statements, expert advice, quality measures, and evidence-based recommendations (Box 1). [1,3] "Clinical Practice Guidelines We Can Trust" is a 290-page publication from the Institute of Medicine. A summary of their "Standards for Developing Trustworthy Clinical Practice Guidelines" appears in Appendix 1 [1,4].

Clinical research: an early barrier

Early barriers to guideline formulation and dissemination are the planning and conduct of the clinical studies that form the bases for guideline development. Clinical research is burdened by a number of impediments including insufficient public participation, information systems, workforce training, and funding (Box 2) [5]. Sung and colleagues [5] contend that solutions to these

Box 1: Criteria for trustworthy guidelines according to the National Academy of Medicine

To be trustworthy, guidelines should:

Be based on a systematic review of the existing evidence

Be developed by a knowledgeable, multidisciplinary panel of experts and representatives from key affected groups

Consider important patient subgroups and patient preferences, as appropriate

Be based on an explicit and transparent process that minimizes distortions, biases, and conflicts of interest

Provide a clear explanation of the logical relationships between alternative care options and health outcomes, and provide ratings of both the quality of evidence and the strength of recommendations

Be reconsidered and revised as appropriate when important new evidence warrants modifications of recommendations

Data from Institute of Medicine (US) Committee on Standards for Developing Trustworthy Clinical Practice Guidelines; Graham R, Mancher M, Miller Wolman D, et al., editors. Clinical Practice Guidelines We Can Trust. Washington (DC): National Academies Press (US); 2011. Available from: https://www.ncbi.nlm.nih.gov/books/NBK209539/ https://doi.org/10.17226/13058

Box 2: Barriers to clinical practice guideline formulation

Translational steps

- Basic science to human studies
- New knowledge to clinical practice and health decision making

Translational blocks

- Lack of willing participants
- Regulatory burden
- Fragmented infrastructure
- Incompatible databases
- Lack of qualified investigators
- Career disincentives
- Practice limitations
- High research costs
- Lack of funding

Intended end point

- Improved health

From Sung NS, Crowley WF, Jr., Genel M, et al. Central challenges facing the national clinical research enterprise. JAMA. 2003;289(10):1278-1287; with permission.

problems are complex and involve the engagement of multiple stakeholders across the entire basic and clinical science research landscape as well as collaboration throughout the spectrum of participants in the health care system.

Cost and time considerations

Adherence to a comprehensive approach for developing guidelines comes at considerable cost. The Institute of Medicine publication cites a cost of $200,000, in 2003 dollars, per individual guideline developed in the United States [1]. An estimate of direct costs for a guideline consensus conference is around $82,000. This estimate does not include costs for other staff or volunteer efforts. The World Health Organization estimates a cost of $100,000 for development of one standard World Health Organization guideline [6].

Some costs for developing guidelines derive from the labor-intensive efforts of collecting, reviewing, evaluating, and collating appropriate published medical literature. Cost increases with the complexity of a topic, the number of pieces of literature reviewed, and the strategies used to complete the process. To establish a guideline for depression, a panel examined more than 90,000 peer-reviewed abstracts [1,7]. The cost and time required to produce a high-quality clinical practice guideline means that remaining current and applicable is an ongoing concern. The World Health Organization estimates that the time to develop a quality guideline can take 9 to 12 months if evidence has been already gathered and as long as 2 to 3 years for guidelines that deal with broad or complicated topics [8].

Conflict of interest

Another issue facing the formulation of clinical practice guidelines is conflict of interest (COI) and its potentially deleterious effects on clinical practice guideline objectivity. Statements to acknowledge and minimize potential COI exist in many methodology manuals for clinical practice guideline formulation [9–11]. A strategy for combatting COI influence has been set forth using the following 3 pillars [12]:

- Place equal emphasis on intellectual and financial conflicts and provide explicit criteria for both.
- A methodologist without important COI should have primary responsibility for each article.
- Experts with important financial or intellectual COI can collect and interpret evidence, but only panel members without important conflicts can be involved in developing the recommendation for a specific question.

Despite guidance from the Institute of Medicine, the problem of relationships with industry continue to plague guideline formulation [13,14].

Differences in grading systems

Different clinical practice guidelines may use different standards by which to assess the quality of evidence found in literature searches. Examples include the Grading of Recommendations Assessment, Development and Evaluation

(GRADE), the Australian National Health and Medical Research Council approach, Formulating Recommendations Matrix, Strength of Recommendation Taxonomy, and the Scottish Intercollegiate Guidelines Network [15–18]. Although these guidelines share similarities, the GRADE system has gained popularity in the last few years [15].

Other barriers to clinical practice guideline formulation

Bias

Clinical practice guidelines are exposed to a high degree of bias. Approximately 75% of clinical studies published in *The Lancet*, the *New England Journal of Medicine*, and the *Journal of the American Medical Association* are industry sponsored. This can become a force multiplier for industry when scores of studies are compiled for inclusion in a clinical practice guideline [1,19].

Generalizability

A shortcoming of many clinical investigations is a lack of generalizability. For example, study participants are often relatively young, healthy, and not representative of many patient subgroups who will be treated using the studied intervention. Those frequently omitted from studies include older patients, those with comorbidities, racial minorities, and the socioeconomically disadvantaged [1,20].

Transparency

Many clinical practice guidelines do not adequately describe the processes used to develop and rate the recommendations they put forward. This shortcoming can have medical as well as legal implications [1,21]. For example, a perceived lack of transparency regarding potential conflicts of interest led to an investigation into the development of Lyme disease guidelines by the Infectious Diseases Society of America [22]. Ultimately, following "multiple meetings, a public hearing, and extensive review of research and other information, the Review Panel concluded that the recommendations contained in the 2006 guidelines were medically and scientifically justified on the basis of all of the available evidence and that no changes to the guidelines were necessary."

Conflicting guidelines and ratings

Conflicting recommendations may result from the use of differing literature search strategies and different evidence grading practices. As many as 70% of guideline developing groups do not reveal the method they use to rate the quality of evidence cited [1].

Implementation and patient outcome measures

Clinical practice guidelines rarely address sufficiently the processes for implementation of their recommendations or the tracking of patient outcomes as a result of guideline-based patient care improvement efforts. Although the words "implement(ation)" and "outcome(s)" may appear in a guideline or their methodology manuals, there are no sections that address implementation planning or patient outcomes measurement [9–11,23].

IMPLEMENTING CLINICAL PRACTICE GUIDELINES

Clinical practice guidelines have historically taken as long as 10 years to achieve even modest levels of adoption [24]. Barriers to the translation of guidelines to practice include the lack of an integrated strategy for implementation, resistance to change, and loss of autonomous decision making. Organizational infrastructure, resource constraints, inadequate support, and cultural factors within and between departments have also emerged as significant barriers to translating guidelines to practice [25]. With this growing awareness, some facilitators to translating guidelines to practice have emerged.

Successful translation of guidelines to practice must consider several variables such as the strength of evidence, superiority over existing practice, and the ease and practicality of trialing and observing the best practice (Table 1) [26–28]. Clinician age, time period of training, and country of training can also influence adoption, because younger clinicians are generally more inclined to modify their practices [29]. A practice setting that fosters improvement in the efficiency and effectiveness of treatments and values social norms can also contribute to more rapid adoption [30,31]. Financial incentives, policies and regulations, and the potential avoidance of litigation have had a variable impact changing physician behavior [32–34]. A hospital's commitment to responding to patient needs also contributes to the

Table 1
Variables affecting adoption of clinical practice guidelines

Guideline qualities	Incentives
Complexity of implementation	Legal
Compatibility with current values	Financial
Trialability of interventions	Overall compensation
Observability of other adopters	Reimbursement for procedures
Advantage over current care	
Individual professional characteristics	Regulation
Age	Accreditation
Country of training	Licensing
Effects on clinical autonomy	
Practice satisfaction	
Concern over health care costs	
Practice setting characteristics	Patient factors
Habit and custom	Demographics
Peer belief systems	Individual patient presentation
Social norms	Compliance patterns
System efficiency	
Implementation support	

Data from Davis DA, Taylor-Vaisey A. Translating guidelines into practice. A systematic review of theoretic concepts, practical experience and research evidence in the adoption of clinical practice guidelines. *CMAJ : Canadian Medical Association journal = journal de l'Association medicale canadienne.* 1997;157(4):408-416 and Rogers EM. Lessons for guidelines from the diffusion of innovations. *The Joint Commission journal on quality improvement.* 1995;21(7):324-328.

implementation of change. For example, a patient population that includes Jehovah's Witnesses may be the driving force for the initiation of a bloodless surgery program, which in turn helps the hospital to support guidelines related to anemia management for all patients.

A summary of barriers and facilitators to guideline adherence are displayed in (Table 2) [35]. Effective implementation of clinical practice guidelines may suffer from multiple barriers, and the use of a single strategy to overcome them may not effective. A separate systematic meta-analysis highlighted a lack of institutional support and patient characteristics as the primary impediments to adoption of, and adherence to, clinical practice guidelines [28].

The complexities of translating guidelines to practice are formidable. The application of implementation science to health care is a recent development and has led to a better understanding of the barriers and facilitators that influence physician decision-making behaviors. Reluctance to modify existing practices, competing guidelines, and institutional culture have all played roles in delaying the adoption of transfusion guidelines [36–38].

Implementation science research focuses on how to translate evidence-based treatments to clinical practice with eventual assessment of outcomes stemming from the application of these treatments to practice [39]. Thus far, the most effective strategies emerging from this work have been audit and feedback, and educational outreach, which have consistently been shown to improve processes and outcomes in a variety of clinical settings [40,41]. Audit and feedback have been particularly helpful in changing physician behavior when individualized, and when practice data are shared in a group setting in a nonpunitive manner [42–47].

Table 2
Barriers and facilitators of guideline adherence

Barriers to Guideline Adherence	Facilitators of Guideline Adherence
Knowledge	Highly effective
Lack of familiarity	Reminder systems
Lack of awareness	Educational outreach
Attitudes	Academic detailing
Lack of agreement with specific clinical practice guidelines	Multiple interventions
	Moderately effective
Lack of agreement with clinical practice guidelines in general	Audit and feedback, especially if:
	Performed concurrently
Lack of outcome expectancy	Provider specific
Lack of elf-efficacy	By peers or opinion leaders
Lack of motivation/inertia of practice	Less effective
Behavior	Lecture-based didactic continuing medical education
External barriers	Mailed, unsolicited materials
Guideline factors	
Environmental factors	

Data from refs[26,28,35]

Peer, practice, and organizational influences

The impact of influential physician peers as levers for promoting change should not be underestimated [41,48]. Pollack and colleagues [49] showed that peer influence is a driver of physician practice styles. They raised the possibility of leveraging this peer influence to limit the adoption and use of low-value care models. Physicians generally respond much better to peer leadership, champions, and data shared from their local practice setting [50]. Physician champions are informal opinion leaders who are well-integrated in the medical community and are respected sources of information who serve as early adopters [51]. They work in similar environments and can influence their peers by serving as models and gatekeepers of information. Their colleagues reach out to them owing to their position, personality, knowledge, influence, and interpersonal skills [52].

Audit and feedback

Audit and feedback are widely used as strategies to improve professional practice, either on their own or as a component of multifaceted quality improvement interventions. In an audit and feedback process, an individual's professional practice or performance is measured and then compared with professional standards or targets. Audit and feedback generally leads to small but potentially important improvements in professional practice. The effectiveness of audit and feedback seems to depend on baseline performance and how the feedback is provided [53]. Factors that positively affect audit and feedback are summarized in Box 3. Audit and feedback is generally most effective when part of a multifaceted approach that includes educational outreach [40,41,54].

Educational outreach

Educational outreach is best performed by physician peers in a multidisciplinary group setting. Alternatively, outside experts can provide concise and relevant information about an approach that has had previous success. These visits should be interactive, provide the practitioner with evidence and rationale

Box 3: Factors positively affecting audit and feedback in changing physician practice

- A significant evidence to practice gap is present at baseline.
- The individual responsible for the audit and feedback is a colleague.
- Serial reporting is completed at regular intervals.
- Audit and feedback is provided for both individual reflection and group discussion.
- Actionable metrics of meaning are selected.

Data from Ivers N, Jamtvedt G, Flottorp S, et al. Audit and feedback: effects on professional practice and healthcare outcomes. *The Cochrane database of systematic reviews.* 2012(6):Cd000259.

for the proposed change, and be an opportunity to discuss any concerns [55]. Soumerai and colleagues [56] showed that a brief, focused educational visit by a transfusion specialist can substantially improve the appropriateness and cost effectiveness of blood product use in surgery.

Academic detailing uses educational outreach experts from outside the institution and has been used to update physicians and support adoption to practice [57,58]. Academic detailing has typically been delivered face to face, but web-based and other technologies are being explored as alternative channels. It has been successfully applied to increase adherence of health care professionals to guidelines for screening [59,60] and to decrease inappropriate use of medicines [26]. Finally, clinical decision support using electronic medical records has been shown to be effective in improving processes of care, with variable effects on improving outcomes [61].

Clinical decision support

Reminders provided at the time and in the context of clinical decision-making can be effective in changing physician behaviors [41]. Whether reminders are provided verbally, on paper, or on a computer screen, they are designed to prompt health professionals to recall relevant information at the point-of-care. Immediate electronic reminders can trigger physicians to adhere to guidelines and therefore assist in behavior change. For example, Schwann and colleagues [62] increased antibiotic administration compliance according to Surgical Care Improvement Project core measures using point-of-care electronic prompts. The use of electronic communication technology provides instantaneous availability of guidelines, which may be particularly crucial for busy physicians [61,63]. This strategy is generally most useful when physicians are in agreement with the information being prompted.

TRANSLATING BLOOD CONSERVATION GUIDELINES TO PRACTICE

There are many guidelines related to perioperative bleeding, coagulopathy, and blood management. The most relevant guidelines with the highest class recommendations are summarized in Table 3 [23,64–66]. Several methods exist to evaluate and describe clinical practice guidelines [67–71]. A critical evaluation of these guidelines falls outside the scope of this review. A simplified framework to aid in comparison of the selected clinical practice guidelines is shown in Table 4.

The experience surrounding the care of patients for cardiac surgery, a clinical area in which there is a high incidence of blood product transfusion, illustrates the shortcomings of focusing solely on guidelines. A publication of blood conservation guidelines developed jointly by The Society of Thoracic Surgeons, the Society of Cardiovascular Anesthesiologists (SCA) and American Society of Extracorporeal Technology was published in 2007 [72], and was assessed using a survey instrument in 2010 [73]. Despite the recommendations, limited adoption had occurred.

Table 3
Guidelines and publication qualities for blood management in cardiac surgery

Category	Society of Thoracic Surgeons/SCA (Ferraris et al, [64] 2011)	EACTS/EACTA (Pagano et al, [23] 2018)	American Society of Anesthesiologists Task Force [65] (2015)	ESA (Kozek-Langenecker et al, [66] 2016)
Publication year	2011	2018	2015	2016
Number of class I recommendations	11	14	16	76[a]
Number of class IIa recommendations	20	17	12	2[b]
Total number of recommendations	35	61	50	153[e]
Class I/IIa: total	88.5%	50.8%	56%	50.9%
Methodology for assessing strength of evidence	AHA/ACCF Task Force on Practice Guidelines Methodology Manual[c]	Scottish Intercollegiate Guidelines Network	Self-developed (specified in guideline text)	GRADE
Guidance for implementation	No	No	No	No
Conflict of interest disclosure	Yes	Yes	No	Yes
Outside review	No	No[d]	Yes	Yes
Summary of recommendations	Yes	No	No	Yes

Abbreviations: ACCF, American College of Cardiology Foundation; AHA, American Heart Association; EACTA, European Association of Cardiothoracic Anesthesiologists; EACTS, European Association for Cardio-Thoracic Surgery; ESA, European Society of Anaesthesiologists.

[a] Includes 1A, 1B, and 1C recommendations.

[b] Additional grade 2 recommendations: 2B = 26, 2C = 110.

[c] http://www.americanheart.org/downloadable/heart/1260477059730 1209Methodology_Manual_for_ACC_AHA_Writing_Committees.pdf.

[d] External review method (Scottish Intercollegiate Guidelines Network).

[e] Does not include statements without a recommendation level but only indication of evidence quality.

Table 4
Class of recommendation/level of evidence by guideline

Category	Society of Thoracic Surgeons/SCA (Ferraris et al [64], 2011)	EACTS/EACTA (Pagano et al [23], 2018)	American Society of Anesthesiologists Task Force [65] (2015)	ESA (Kozek-Langenecker et al [66], 2017)[m]
Stop antiplatelet and/ or anticoagulants preoperatively	I(B)	IIa(B) – DAPT IIa(C) – DOAC	A2-E[f] B1-E[g]	1C
Evaluation/treatment of preoperative anemia	IIa (B)	IIa(B)[a] IIb(C)[b]	A1-B[h]	1C
Blood management or conservation program	IIa (B)	I (C)	A2-E	N/C[n]
Intraoperative antifibrinolytic therapy	I(A)	I (A)	A1-B	1A
Low volume cardiopulmonary bypass circuit	I(A)	IIA(B)	N/C	N/C
Acute normovolemic hemodilution	IIb(B)	IIb(B)	A1-B	2C
Retrograde autologous priming	IIb(B)	IIa(A)	N/C	N/C
Modified ultrafiltration	N/C	IIb(B)	N/C	N/C
Intraoperative cell salvage	IIa(A)	IIa(B)	N/C	1B
Restrictive transfusion/ use of transfusion triggers	IIa	I (B)[d] IIb(B)[e]	A1-B[i] A2-E[j]	1A
Use of transfusion guideline/algorithm	I (A)	IIA(B)	A2-B[l]	1B
POC hemostatic/ viscoelastic testing	I (A)	III(C)[c]	A1-B[k] A2-B[l]	1C

Abbreviations: DAPT, dual antiplatelet therapy; DOAC, direct acting oral anticoagulant; EACTA, European Association of Cardiothoracic Anesthesiologists; EACTS, European Association for Cardio-Thoracic Surgery; ESA, European Society of Anaesthesiologists; N/C, no comment in the guideline.

[a] Erythropoietin with iron for non–iron deficiency anemia.
[b] Oral or intravenous iron for mildly or severely anemic patients.
[c] POC testing not recommended.
[d] Packed red blood cell transfusion based on clinical condition versus fixed hemoglobin threshold.
[e] Hematocrit of 21% to 24% during cardiopulmonary bypass is adequate if the DO_2 is maintained.
[f] Discontinue aspirin preoperatively.
[g] Bridge warfarin with low-molecular-weight heparin.
[h] Erythropoietin with or without iron.
[i] Fewer red blood cell transfusions.
[j] Equivocal findings for mortality, cardiac, neurologic or pulmonary complications, and hospital length of stay.
[k] Thromboelastography versus standard coagulation testing.
[l] Rotational thromboelastometry-guided algorithm versus no algorithm.
[m] Entries without grade of recommendation excluded.
[n] No specific recommendation is given regarding a patient blood management program. Patient blood management programs are referenced in different sections (eg, anemia management).

USE OF AN IMPLEMENTATION SCIENCE-BASED APPROACH

Until recently, effective strategies for bridging the evidence-to-practice gap in health care have been largely underused [74,75]. Implementation science focuses on identifying and targeting factors that are critical for successful implementation. It seeks to "understand factors that determine why an evidence-based intervention may or may not be adopted within specific health care or public health settings and uses this information to develop and test strategies to improve the speed, quantity and quality of uptake" [76]. Implementation science-based approaches have the potential to translate evidence-based patient blood management into practice.

The application of implementation science requires an appreciation of 3 key principles (Table 5) [77]. First is the appreciation of the importance of changing the behaviors of clinicians, patients, and policymakers. Most change strategies are designed to improve the capability, opportunity, and motivation of the affected individuals. For patient blood management, this means knowing the guidelines, having ready access to the clinical and laboratory data needed to make transfusion decisions, and believing that one can influence changes in practice. Second is the need to engage a wide range of stakeholders whose influence is imperative to achieving sustained improvements in outcomes. In addition to frontline physicians, this group includes blood bank leadership and institutional executives, because the change strategies likely require alterations to process and policy as well as to priorities and resources. Finally, the physician leader or champion must be flexible and willing to tolerate the iterative and nonlinear nature of the process of addressing barriers and discovering the enablers needed to adapt guidelines to the real-world situation.

In many cases, a readiness assessment conducted before an intervention reveal conditions or behaviors (mediators) that need to be incorporated into implementation strategy. For patient blood management, a systematic,

Table 5
Essential principles in implementation science

Principle	Change strategies
Focus on changing provider behaviors	COM-B model Capability/opportunity/motivation Plus behavior change wheel
Engage all stakeholders affected by new intervention or behavior	Community-engaged research Individuals (patients and providers) Delivery (health system) Others (government, regulators)
Provide flexible commitment to implementation	Iterative, cyclical processes Long-term planning and expectations

Abbreviation: COM-C, capability, opportunity, motivation and behaviour.

Data from Handley MA, Gorukanti A, Cattamanchi A. Strategies for implementing implementation science: a methodological overview. Emergency medicine journal: EMJ. 2016;33(9):660-664

step-by-step process should include 3 major phases. The preimplementation or planning phase starts with making the case for the implementation strategy by clearly establishing its relation to a health problem. Once assembled, the case can be further improved as the leadership team makes stakeholder rounds. Their presentation should delineate the performance gap (between the current and the ideal practice or behavior) and the outcome gap (between the current and the expected health outcomes). For blood conservation, the performance gap will likely be unnecessary blood transfusions with an outcome gap of reduced safety, effectiveness, and patient centeredness. The intervention or behavior change might be adherence to a point-of-care (POC)-driven transfusion algorithm.

Designing the implementation strategy is the next phase and should focus on identifying mediators that represent barriers and facilitators of the desired behavior change. In the case of a POC-driven transfusion algorithm, examples of barriers include availability of laboratory analyzers at the point of care, increased cost of tests and personnel, as well as the risk of being cited for noncompliance (of an ancillary site) by external regulatory agencies. Examples of enablers would be support from a multidisciplinary change team with performance reviews and shared goals supported by the chief operating officer. Careful selection of the implementation strategy is critical, and guidance by experts in quality improvement, human factors and/or implementation science are recommended [78].

Finally, evaluate the implementation strategy by assessing:

1. The process: Is it acceptable and feasible?
2. The mediators of change: Do components modify targeted barriers and enhance targeted enablers?
3. The outcomes: How do they affect the institution (eg, reduced transfusions, cost) and patients (eg, reduced morbidity)?

The design and evaluation of an implementation strategy for increasing adherence to a POC-driven transfusion algorithm in the operating room is shown in Table 6, and a similar display for approaching preoperative anemia management is summarized is shown in Table 7. Additional support and resources that can be used to help close the evidence-to-practice gap are summarized in Table 8.

IMPLEMENTATION STRATEGY FOR PATIENT BLOOD MANAGEMENT

The Society for the Advancement of Patient Blood Management defines patient blood management as "the timely application of evidence-based medical and surgical concepts designed to maintain hemoglobin concentration, optimize hemostasis, and minimize blood loss in an effort to improve patient outcomes" [88]. Implementation of a patient blood management program requires significant collaboration between clinicians and administrators. These programs touch almost every specialty in medicine. A transfusion specialist plays a key

Table 6
Evaluating implementation strategy for a transfusion algorithm

Performance gap	Unnecessary blood transfusions gap between current and ideal practice/behavior	
Outcome gap	Reduced safety, effectiveness, and patient-centeredness gap between current and expected health outcomes	
Intervention (behavior change)	Adhere to POC-driven transfusion algorithm in the operating room	
Process	*Dimension*	*Measurement*
Acceptability	Transfusion triggers	Survey, focus group discussions
Feasibility	Laboratory TAT	% of sample TAT of <5–10 min
Fidelity	Transfusion algorithm	% protocol adherence
Mediators		
Modify barriers	POC analyzers CLIA/CAP certification Net cost of intervention	Yes/no analyzer in OR # CAP citations per inspection Yes/no hospital ROI determination
Enhance enabler	Multidisciplinary patient blood management team performance review Collective discussion of results	Yes/no presence of unit-based team Number of audit and feedback per year Number of group conferences per year
Outcomes		
Transfusions	Restrictive transfusion	Percent transfused Units per 1000 patient-days
Cost	Operating margin	AP-DRG-adjusted direct costs
Safety	Patient	Risk-adjusted morbidity

Abbreviations: AP-DRG, all patient-diagnosis related groups; CAP, College of American Pathologists; CLIA, Clinical Laboratory Improvement Amendments; POC, point of care; TAT, turnaround time.

role in the coordination of multiple different specialties (medical and surgical) as well as laboratory and nonclinical staff.

The first national patient blood management program was implemented in Australia following the World Health Assembly's resolution WHA63.12 [89]. Australia adopted the "3 pillar model" of optimizing red cell mass: minimizing blood loss and bleeding and optimizing physiologic reserve to anemia. Guidelines were developed in 6 modules, including critical bleeding and massive transfusion, perioperative, medical, intensive care, obstetrics, and pediatrics and neonates. Other countries, including the UK, Spain, and Switzerland, have established similar programs.

The Simplified International Recommendations for the Implementation of Patient Blood Management described by Meybohm and colleagues [79] recommends the use of bundles to improve adoption. Bundles are "a straightforward set of evidenced-based interventions for a defined patient population that, when implemented together, will result in significantly better, more penetrating and sustainable outcomes than when implemented individually" [90]. Broken down into separate "blocks," an individual hospital can more easily determine

Table 7
Evaluating implementation strategy for preoperative anemia management

Performance Gap	Avoidable red blood cell transfusions gap between current and ideal practice/behavior	
Outcome Gap	Reduced safety, effectiveness, and patient-centeredness gap between current and expected health outcomes	
Intervention (behavior change)	Active management of preoperative anemia	
Process	*Dimension*	*Measurement*
Acceptability	Patients and surgeons	Survey, focus group discussion
Feasibility	Cost and logistics	Yes/no approved clinical pathway
Fidelity	Treatment algorithm	Percent protocol adherence
Mediators		
Modify barriers	Patient inconvenience Reimbursement by payer Care coordination Net cost of intervention	Number of additional patient visits Yes/no hospital ROI determination Yes/no part of preoperative process Yes/no hospital ROI determination
Enhance enabler	Bloodless surgery program	Number of referrals for program
Outcomes		
Untreated anemia	Anemia on morning of surgery	Percent with preoperative anemia
Transfusion	Red blood cells	Red blood cells per 1000 patient-days
Cost	Moderate/severe anemia on discharge	Readmission rate
Safety	Patient	Risk-adjusted morbidity

Abbreviation: ROI, return on investment.

which components would be most realistic and beneficial to implement (Table 9).

Block 1 of recommendations by Meybohm and colleagues includes a patient blood management project manager with a "central role in charge of communication, education, and documentation" who continually informs hospital administrators and medical staff. They also recommend an education program that includes standard operating procedures, clinical protocols, and checklists. Block 2 begins with anemia management, which includes early identification of anemic patients and those undergoing operations with greater than a 10% probability of transfusion and optimization of red cell mass. Block 3 ensures optimization of hemostasis. Before red blood cell transfusion, the use of a coagulation algorithm in accordance with local standards and practice should be adopted. Block 4 introduces a multidisciplinary approach to blood conservation. This approach consists of early anemia detection, restricted laboratory testing with small phlebotomy volumes, and decreasing waste volume. Block 5 focuses

Table 8
Additional support and resources

Source	Content
Agency for Healthcare Quality and Research (AHRQ website) [2]	Formation of unit-based safety programs
American College of Cardiology and American Heart Association (Chan 2017) [41].	Clinical practice guideline implementation strategies
Meybohm et al [79], 2017	Implementation strategy for patient blood management
Proctor et al [80], 2011	Measuring implementation outcomes
Greilich et al [81], 2018	Diffusing successful pilots
Frank et al [82], 2017	System-wide spread of patient blood management
Haynes et al [83], 2017; and Haugen et al [84], 2019	Use of implementation-based approach to reducing mortality using surgical checklists
Journal of Implementation Science [85] (https://implementationscience.biomedcentral.com)	General resources
Annual Conference on the Science of Dissemination and Implementation in Health [86] (https://www.academyhealth.org/events)	General resources
UCSF Department of Epidemiology and Biostatistics [87] (https://epibiostat.ucsf.edu/certificate-programs)	Online training programs in implementation science for leaders in quality improvement

on optimal resource management, particularly adopting a restrictive transfusion practice. Emphasis on single-unit transfusion and specification of indications for transfusion help reduce overall transfusion. Block 6 is benchmarking. Data should be collected on all aspects of a patient blood management program, both administrative and clinical. Data can be reported by service line as well as by individuals. The adoption of bundles facilitates implementation of patient blood management programs in a stepwise fashion without requiring immediate major changes that may not be well-received.

Support from executives, at the hospital and system levels, is imperative for a patient blood management program's success [81]. Also imperative is using a clinical community approach, consisting of physician-led, self-governing stakeholders to improve quality in health care. The Johns Hopkins Health System adopted a patient blood management program across 5 hospitals [82]. The largest hospital in the system, The Johns Hopkins Hospital, began an educational program in each department. Focusing on abundant high-quality evidence, an educational program initially targeted surgical services and transfusion triggers and thresholds. Data acquisition was initially provided via a commercial system (IMPACT Online, Haemonetics Corp, Braintree, MA). Equally important to the clinical education component was a formal business plan that included salary support for transfusion specialists (including 1

Table 9
Summary of blood management bundles

Block 1	
Patient blood management project management	Patient blood management stakeholder involvement Education Local standards of practice/protocols
Block 2	
Manage patient's anemia	Preoperative management of anemia (subgroup of surgical patients) Improve cardiovascular and pulmonary tolerance of anemia Anemia management in postoperative/hospitalized patients
Block 3	
Optimizing coagulopathy	Preoperative management of coagulopathy Hemostasis management in hospitalized patients
Block 4	
Interdisciplinary blood conservation modalities	Reduction of diagnostic-associated blood loss Reduction of surgery-related blood loss (subgroup of surgical patients)
Block 5	
Optimal blood use with patient-centered decision making	Patient-centered decision making
Block 6	
Patient blood management-related metrics, patient's outcome, benchmark	Patient blood management–related metrics Patient's outcome Benchmarking Program budget for patient blood management Hospital audit for patient blood management Hospital accreditation for patient blood management

Data from Meybohm P, Richards T, Isbister J, et al. Patient Blood Management Bundles to Facilitate Implementation. Transfusion medicine reviews. 2017;31(1):62-71.

anesthesiologist), a nurse coordinator, and a data manager. Peer comparison was accomplished with rank-order bar graphs with individual identifiers available within departments but not between departments. Blood acquisition cost savings were $2,102,273 per year, a 400% return on investment.

HIGH OPPORTUNITY AREAS FOR PERIOPERATIVE BLOOD CONSERVATION: LESSONS FROM CARDIAC SURGERY

Although much of the evidence base discussed in this article derives from cardiac surgery, the broader goal is to provide a framework for translating guidelines to an improved practice of perioperative blood conservation for patients with anemia and/or patients at risk for at least moderate blood loss (>500 mL).

Implementation of a preoperative anemia management program

Anemia is a predictor of long-term mortality in patients undergoing cardiac surgery (Fig. 1) [91–95]. It is also an independent risk factor for postoperative

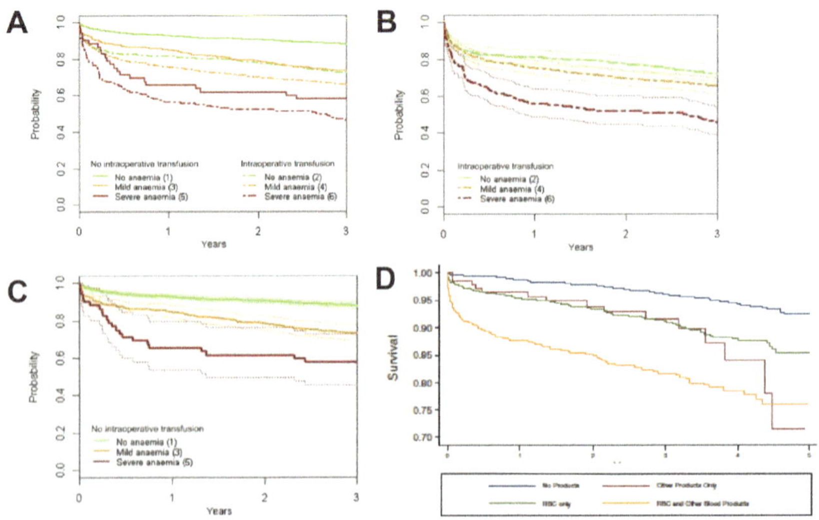

Fig. 1. Association of transfusion of blood and blood products with long-term survival. (*A, B*) Anemia severity, transfusion, and survival. (*C*) Anemia severity and survival. (*D*) Transfusion and survival. ([*A–C*] *From* von Heymann C, Kaufner L, Sander M, et al. Does the severity of preoperative anemia or blood transfusion have a stronger impact on long-term survival after cardiac surgery? *The Journal of Thoracic and Cardiovascular Surgery.* 2016;152(5):1412-1420; with permission. [*D*] *From* Bhaskar B, Dulhunty J, Mullany DV, Fraser JF. Impact of blood product transfusion on short and long-term survival after cardiac surgery: more evidence. *The Annals of Thoracic Surgery.* 2012;94(2):460-467.)

renal dysfunction, stroke, and prolonged hospital length of stay [93]. Although there are conflicting data, preoperative administration of erythropoietin plus iron or a single dose of erythropoietin, have been shown to reduce transfusion requirements, improve survival, and shorten hospital length of stay [96,97]. This management program can stand alone or be part of a larger, institution-wide patient blood management bundle as recently described by Meybohm and colleagues [79].

The initial step in establishing such a program requires assessing the institutional need for decreasing transfusion rates in cardiac surgery. Gathering information about the number of anemic patients undergoing surgery and transfusion rates for those with varying degrees of anemia and their outcomes can help an institution assess the potential impact of an anemia management program. These data can be collected from enterprise databases and clinical registries such as the Society of Thoracic Surgeons National Database. After determining whether a cardiac surgical program would benefit from a preoperative anemia management program, the next phase is to conduct an assessment of readiness, which includes a determination of feasibility and acceptability of a program proposal. Resources vary among hospital systems, and it is advisable to survey the availability of infrastructure, funding, personnel, equipment, and other services (ie, laboratory, pharmacy) necessary for successful implementation. Based on the initial investigations into the feasibility of a project, realistic goals or milestones should be determined. Even if a comprehensive preoperative anemia program may not be possible, elements of the program may still be implemented on a smaller scale.

Development of a management team and engagement with stakeholders

Successful implementation of a preoperative anemia management program requires a central management team to coordinate patient selection, determine treatment pathways, and evaluate quality outcomes such as transfusion rates and perioperative adverse events. This management team also needs to engage with hospital leadership and primary stakeholders, including patients, surgeons, anesthesiologists, hematologists, blood bank personnel, laboratory medicine leadership, and perioperative physicians. It is critical that the benefits to patients and the cost-to-benefit ratio be emphasized to all major stakeholders and hospital leaders. The cost effectiveness of anemia management programs has been shown for patients with chronic kidney disease, and recent simulations of patient blood management bundles have revealed the potential for reduced hospital length of stay and associated cost savings. Leadership awareness and support are crucial to overcoming barriers to implementation of an anemia treatment program.

Planning the intervention

Factors important for designing an anemia treatment program are summarized in Table 10 and include patient eligibility criteria, the treatment regimen, overall cost, monitoring for patient safety, and performance evaluation. Patients referred for cardiac surgery can be flagged for predetermined hemoglobin or hematocrit levels. The level at which significant anemia is defined can be either an institutional decision or based on national and international guidelines. Once a patient is identified with preoperative anemia, it is important for the preoperative clinical staff to investigate the cause of the anemia.

Treatment pathway

Although oral iron supplementation is the most common treatment for iron deficiency anemia, normalization of hemoglobin levels can take weeks [98]. Intravenous iron supplementation can improve hemoglobin levels safely and more rapidly than oral supplements, making it more appropriate in the context of cardiac surgery [99]. Intravenous iron therapy needs to be administered and monitored by health care professionals, which may lead to increased cost and facility use. Using hospital outpatient chemotherapy infusion centers may help to decrease costs and, in some systems, provide a source of revenue. Patients with coagulopathies, a history of stroke, or hypersensitivity to intravenous iron should be excluded from this treatment.

A recent meta-analysis found that preoperative erythropoietin treatment for anemia in cardiac surgical patients leads to a 50% decrease in the incidence of perioperative blood transfusions [100]. In addition, preoperative administration

Table 10
Factors important for designing an anemia management program

Factors	Special Considerations
Patient eligibility criteria	Level of anemia (hemoglobin or hematocrit) Underlying causes of anemia Identification of patients
Treatment regimen	Treatment (iron and/or erythropoietin) Timing and duration of treatment Surveillance of patients (follow-up visits and tests)
Cost of implementation	Medications Laboratory tests Staffing Identification and follow-up of patients (clinic?)
Monitoring for patient safety	Side effects Complications Rate of increase of hemoglobin
Performance evaluation of program	Cost Acceptance of program Number of patients screened Number of patients screened Annual transfusion rates Other outcomes

of erythropoietin with iron has been shown to be as safe as iron therapy alone in a variety of surgical populations including cardiothoracic surgery [101]. Dosing regimens vary and even ultrashort courses (0–5 days) of erythropoietin with or without intravenous iron have been shown to be effective [96,97,102,103]. Some treatment regimens include postoperative doses of erythropoietin during patient hospitalization. Scheduling and logistical barriers may make it difficult to adhere to established treatment regimens, so shorter courses may be preferable.

Strategy for surveillance and monitoring

Previous experience in patients with chronic kidney disease provides a framework for monitoring erythropoietin therapy [104–106]. Regardless of the dose or administration schedule, erythropoietin therapy should be accompanied by formal monitoring for the development of venous thrombosis or pulmonary embolism. It is recommended to use venous thromboembolism prophylaxis during erythropoietin therapy. Contraindications to erythropoietin treatment include known malignancy, significant hypertension, thrombophilia, or a high risk of stroke. Although the risks of parenteral iron administration have been reduced with new iron formulations, the risks of anaphylaxis, thrombosis, or iron overload still exist. During the preoperative treatment period, the patient should have 1 to 2 visits for surveillance of side effects or adverse events. The rate of increase in hemoglobin should not exceed 1 g/dL per week. Diastolic blood pressures should not exceed 100 mm Hg. Therapy should also be halted in those patients who display allergic reactions or complications at any time during the course of treatment.

Infrastructure and cost

Major costs include laboratory studies, cost of medications, and hospital or clinic staff. Facilities should be able to provide space and equipment for the intravenous administration of iron. For example, in 2015 at the University of Texas Southwestern Medical Center in Dallas, the average anemic patient undergoing cardiac surgery received 3.07 units of packed red blood cells, compared with 1.3 units for nonanemic patients. These anemic patients also had longer ICU stays resulting in an average additional cost of $10,282. Acquisition cost of 1 unit of packed red blood cells is $155. However, the total cost of packed red blood cells units may be as much as 4 times higher owing to costs associated with testing, storage, administration and complications [88]. The cost of an EPOGEN (Amgen, Thousand Oaks, CA) injection plus FERAHEME (AMAG Pharmaceuticals, Waltham, MA) for an 80-kg patient is about $2232. If preoperative anemia therapy is instituted, the predicted cost savings may approach $8000 per patient.

Performance evaluation

When initiating any quality improvement or treatment program, it is important to develop methods to test performance. It is also important to evaluate how well the program is implemented at set intervals after program initiation. Stakeholder acceptance of a blood conservation program can be measured through feedback surveys, a feedback hotline or website, and interval group feedback sessions, particularly of the major clinical providers (cardiac surgeons, cardiac anesthesiologists, critical care physicians, and the perioperative and intensive care unit staff). Adoption of the program can be measured with a variety of methods, including a review of pharmacy administration logs for erythropoietin and parenteral iron supplementation, a count of patients referred for anemia treatment, and a system for reporting staff use. Reevaluation on a monthly basis is recommended after program implementation to assess for areas of waste or possible avenues for improvement. Finally, penetration of the program can be calculated by looking at the number of anemic cardiac surgical patients enrolled in the treatment program divided by the total number of anemic cardiac surgical patients diagnosed or screened in the preoperative setting.

At some point after a program has been implemented, service metrics should be evaluated. In the case of blood conservation, the service metrics are well-defined. Annual transfusion rates in cardiac surgery cases (typically excluding aortic surgery, ventricular assist devices, transplants, or other procedures with very high blood loss) should be monitored. Other variables that should be recorded include preoperative and postoperative complication including prolonged ventilation, stroke, acute kidney injury, renal failure, infection, sepsis, and death. Length of stay, cost of care, and staff work-hours can also be used. The metrics should be analyzed with reference to clinical providers including surgeon and anesthesiologist. Results of the analysis can hopefully provide enough data to indicate the cost benefit and/or outcomes benefit of the program.

USE OF A SURVEY INSTRUMENT TO DRIVE LOCAL AND NATIONAL PERIOPERATIVE BLOOD CONSERVATION

As described elsewhere in this article, audit and feedback is one of the most reliable methods for improving process and clinical outcomes. Surveys have long been used to collect, compare, and analyze information from either the general population or targeted groups. A well-designed questionnaire can provide valid and actionable information about behaviors, practices, and unjustified variations in practices. One approach in quality improvement is the use of a survey as a mechanism for audit and feedback. Audit and feedback methods have been shown to be useful tools in implementation science to promote the adoption of clinical recommendations or consensus policies [41]. Surveys can evaluate the efficacy of particular clinical interventions, identify knowledge gaps among providers and reveal impediments to adoption of best clinical practices. Surveys performed by the American Society of Anesthesiologists Committee on Transfusion Medicine in 1981 and 2002 have been used to demonstrate notable reductions in hemoglobin triggers, increased use of POC coagulation testing, and increased availability of autologous blood salvage equipment [107]. Previously mentioned was the clinical practice guideline for blood conservation published in 2007 [37,73,108,109]. Although both surveys provided useful information, the prolonged interval between surveys and lack of serial data limited their usefulness as instruments for audit and feedback. The biennial hospital survey on patient safety created by the Agency for Healthcare Research and Quality is more representative of how a validated survey might be used for audit and feedback for patient blood management [110].

Survey instruments can also be used by medical societies to support the development of quality metrics and champion efforts to close evidence-to-practice gaps. For example, the SCA, American Society of Anesthesiologists, and Anesthesia Quality Institute's (AQI) recently created a metric for blood conservation during cardiopulmonary bypass (AQI49). The 4 components of this composite metric include the (1) use of lysine analogues, (2) use of minicircuits, retrograde autologous priming, ultrafiltration, (3) use of red cell salvage, and (4) use of a transfusion algorithm with POC testing [111]. This composite metric has been added to the AQI's Qualified Clinical Data Registry and has provisional acceptance by the National Quality Forum as an allowable measure for merit-based incentive payment system. Concurrent with this work, the SCA Blood Conservation Work Group designed a serial survey instrument for audit and feedback both locally and nationally. The potential role of a serial survey in translating guidelines to practice is shown in Fig. 2. The survey addresses (1) preoperative preparation, (2) intraoperative techniques, (3) transfusion avoidance and algorithms, (4) POC testing, (5) hemostatic agents and factor concentrates, and (6) massive bleeding and transfusion. Locally, a serial survey could

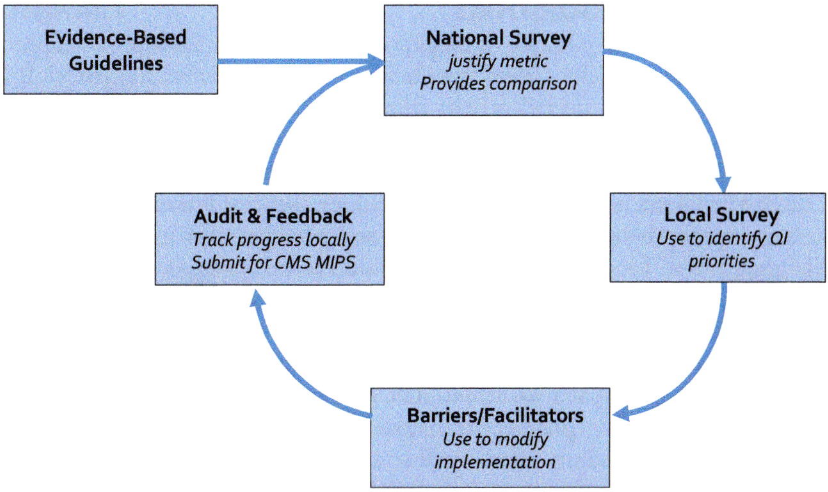

Fig. 2. Role of SCA serial blood conservation survey in support of efforts to translate guidelines to practice. CMS, Centers for Medicare and Medicaid Services; MIPS, merit-based incentive payment system; NQF, National Quality Foundation; QI, quality improvement; SCA, Society of Cardiovascular Anesthesiologists.

be tailored for use as an audit and feedback tool focusing on their greatest priority. Comparative data from the national survey (conducted every 2–4 years) could be used help local champions with policymakers and promote a common language among a peer-to-peer collaboration. Aligning local, regional, and national efforts has the potential to increase the capacity and effectiveness of blood conservation champions. The 2017 SCA Survey of Blood Conservation in Cardiac Surgery had 525 respondents. It demonstrated the AQI49 composite is justified, because fewer than 30% of the practices reported conformance with all 4 components. Although low, the National Quality Forum prefers metrics supported by Class I evidence with large evidence-to-practice gaps. In the beginning, top decile performance could be as low 40% to 60% until wider adoption occurs.

Although survey research does have some inherent difficulties, including assessing the validity of the survey data, assessing for the presence of survey bias, and acquiring adequate response rates, a survey is a relatively simple and cost-effective tool to help promote and assess the implementation of quality standards in health care [112]. The designation of local champions, working in conjunction with regional and national efforts to provide meaningful metric and comparative data, is essential. The maintenance of survey response rates should ideally be more than 30% to maintain validity of the audit and feedback system. The development of a peer-to-peer network capable of sharing barriers and facilitators to perioperative blood conservation is vital to program success.

Available at: https://www.acc.org//~/media/Non-Clinical/Files-PDFs-Excel-MS-Word-etc/Guidelines/About%20Guidelines%20and%20Clinical%20Documents/Methodology/2014/Methodology%20Practice%20Guidelines.pdf. Accessed February, 11, 2019.
[11] American College of Cardiology Foundation. Manual for ACCF clinical expert consensus documents writing committees 2008. Available at: https://www.acc.org/~/media/Non-Clinical/Files-PDFs-Excel-MS-Wordetc/Guidelines/About%20Guidelines%20and%20Clinical%20Documents/Methodology/2014/Methodology%20Expert%20Consensus%20Documents.pdf?la=en. Accessed March, 13, 2019.
[12] Guyatt G, Akl EA, Hirsh J, et al. The vexing problem of guidelines and conflict of interest: a potential solution. Ann Intern Med 2010;152(11):738–41.
[13] Mendelson TB, Meltzer M, Campbell EG, et al. Conflicts of interest in cardiovascular clinical practice guidelines. Arch Intern Med 2011;171(6):577–84.
[14] Kung J, Miller RR, Mackowiak PA. Failure of clinical practice guidelines to meet institute of medicine standards: two more decades of little, if any, progress. Arch Intern Med 2012;172(21):1628–33.
[15] Kredo T, Bernhardsson S, Machingaidze S, et al. Guide to clinical practice guidelines: the current state of play. Int J Qual Health Care 2016;28(1):122–8.
[16] Ebell MH, Siwek J, Weiss BD, et al. Strength of recommendation taxonomy (SORT): a patient-centered approach to grading evidence in the medical literature. J Am Board Fam Pract 2004;17(1):59–67.
[17] Guyatt GH, Oxman AD, Vist GE, et al. GRADE: an emerging consensus on rating quality of evidence and strength of recommendations. BMJ 2008;336(7650):924–6.
[18] Scottish Intercollegiate Guidelines Network. SIGN 50: a guideline developer's handbook. Available at: https://www.sign.ac.uk/assets/sign50_2015.pdf. Accessed March, 11, 2019.
[19] House of Commons Health Committee. The influence of the pharmaceutical industry. 2005. Available at: https://publications.parliament.uk/pa/cm200405/cmselect/cmhealth/42/42.pdf. Accessed March, 13, 2019.
[20] Brown A. Clinical practice guidelines: implications for vulnerable patients: development of geriatric diabetes guidelines. Paper presented at the IOM Committee on Standards for Developing Trustworthy Clinical Practice Guidelines meeting. Washington, DC, January 11, 2010.
[21] Lantos PM, Charini WA, Medoff G, et al. Final report of the Lyme disease review panel of the Infectious Diseases Society of America. Clin Infect Dis 2010;51(1):1–5.
[22] Attorney general says today's IDSA hearing should set standard for establishing medical guidelines [press release] Washington, D.C. Available at: https://portal.ct.gov/AG/Press-Releases-Archived/2009-Press-Releases/Attorney-General-Says-Todays-IDSA-Hearing-Should-Set-Standard-For-Establishing-Medical-Guidelines. Accessed June 17, 2019.
[23] Pagano D, Milojevic M, Meesters MI, et al. 2017 EACTS/EACTA guidelines on patient blood management for adult cardiac surgery. Eur J Cardiothoracic Surg 2018;53(1):79–111.
[24] Balas EA, Boren SA. Managing clinical knowledge for health care improvement. Yearb Med Inform 2000;(1):65–70.
[25] Vander Schaaf EB, Seashore CJ, Randolph GD. Translating clinical guidelines into practice: challenges and opportunities in a dynamic health care environment. North Carolina Med J 2015;76(4):230–4.
[26] Davis DA, Taylor-Vaisey A. Translating guidelines into practice. A systematic review of theoretic concepts, practical experience and research evidence in the adoption of clinical practice guidelines. CMAJ 1997;157(4):408–16.
[27] Rogers EM. Lessons for guidelines from the diffusion of innovations. Jt Comm J Qual 1995;21(7):324–8.

[28] Francke AL, Smit MC, de Veer AJ, et al. Factors influencing the implementation of clinical guidelines for health care professionals: a systematic meta-review. BMC Med Inform Decis Mak 2008;8:38.
[29] Ferrier BM, Woodward CA, Cohen M, et al. Clinical practice guidelines. New-to-practice family physicians' attitudes. Can Fam Physician 1996;42:463–8.
[30] Conroy M, Shannon W. Clinical guidelines: their implementation in general practice. Br J Gen Pract 1995;45(396):371–5.
[31] Ellrodt AG, Conner L, Riedinger M, et al. Measuring and improving physician compliance with clinical practice guidelines. A controlled interventional trial. Ann Intern Med 1995;122(4):277–82.
[32] Robinson MB. Evaluation of medical audit. J Epidemiol Community Health 1994;48(5): 435–40.
[33] Jutras D. Clinical practice guidelines as legal norms. CMAJ 1993;148(6):905–8.
[34] Borowitz M, Sheldon T. Controlling health care: from economic incentives to micro-clinical regulation. Health Econ 1993;2(3):201–4.
[35] Cabana MD, Rand CS, Powe NR, et al. Why don't physicians follow clinical practice guidelines? A framework for improvement. JAMA 1999;282(15):1458–65.
[36] Qian F, Osler TM, Eaton MP, et al. Variation of blood transfusion in patients undergoing major noncardiac surgery. Ann Surg 2013;257(2):266–78.
[37] Bennett Guerrero E, Zhao Y, O'Brien SM, et al. Variation in use of blood transfusion in coronary artery bypass graft surgery. JAMA 2010;304(14):1568–75.
[38] Cote C, MacLeod JB, Yip AM, et al. Variation in transfusion rates within a single institution: exploring the effect of differing practice patterns on the likelihood of blood product transfusion in patients undergoing cardiac surgery. J Thorac Cardiovasc Surg 2015;149(1): 297–302.
[39] Khoury MJ, Gwinn M, Yoon PW, et al. The continuum of translation research in genomic medicine: how can we accelerate the appropriate integration of human genome discoveries into health care and disease prevention? Genet Med 2007;9(10):665–74.
[40] Grimshaw JM, Shirran L, Thomas R, et al. Changing provider behavior: an overview of systematic reviews of interventions. Med Care 2001;39(8 Suppl 2):Ii2–45.
[41] Chan WV, Pearson TA, Bennett GC, et al. ACC/AHA special report: clinical practice guideline implementation strategies: a summary of systematic reviews by the NHLBI implementation science work group: a report of the American College of Cardiology/American Heart Association Task Force on Clinical Practice Guidelines. Circulation 2017;135(9): e122–37.
[42] Harvey PA, Murphy MC, Dornom E, et al. Implementing evidence-based guidelines: inpatient management of chronic obstructive pulmonary disease. Intern Med J 2005;35(3): 151–5.
[43] Baker R, Falconer Smith J, Lambert PC. Randomised controlled trial of the effectiveness of feedback in improving test ordering in general practice. Scand J Prim Health Care 2003;21(4):219–23.
[44] Goff DC Jr, Massing MW, Bertoni AG, et al. Enhancing quality of heart failure care in managed Medicare and Medicaid in North Carolina: results of the North Carolina Achieving Cardiac Excellence (NC ACE) Project. Am Heart J 2005;150(4):717–24.
[45] Bradley EH, Holmboe ES, Mattera JA, et al. Data feedback efforts in quality improvement: lessons learned from US hospitals. Qual Saf Health Care 2004;13(1):26–31.
[46] Leung K, Su S, Morris MW. When is criticism not constructive? The roles of fairness perceptions and dispositional attributions in employee acceptance of critical supervisory feedback. Hum Relat 2001;54(9):1155–87.
[47] DeShon RP, Kozlowski SW, Schmidt AM, et al. A multiple-goal, multilevel model of feedback effects on the regulation of individual and team performance. J Appl Psychol 2004;89(6):1035–56.

[48] Lomas J, Enkin M, Anderson GM, et al. Opinion leaders vs audit and feedback to implement practice guidelines. Delivery after previous cesarean section. JAMA 1991;265(17):2202–7.
[49] Pollack CE, Soulos PR, Herrin J, et al. The impact of social contagion on physician adoption of advanced imaging tests in breast cancer. J Natl Cancer Inst 2017;109(8).
[50] Dopson S, Locock L, Gabbay J, et al. Evidence-based medicine and the implementation gap. Health 2003;7(3):311–30.
[51] Greer AL. The state of the art versus the state of the science. The diffusion of new medical technologies into practice. Int J Technol Assess Health Care 1988;4(1):5–26.
[52] Wenrich JW, Mann FC, Morris WC, et al. Informal educators for practicing physicians. J Med Educ 1971;46(4):299–305.
[53] Ivers N, Jamtvedt G, Flottorp S, et al. Audit and feedback: effects on professional practice and healthcare outcomes. Cochrane Database Syst Rev 2012;(6) Cd000259.
[54] Bero LA, Grilli R, Grimshaw JM, et al. Closing the gap between research and practice: an overview of systematic reviews of interventions to promote the implementation of research findings. The Cochrane Effective Practice and Organization of Care Review Group. BMJ 1998;317(7156):465–8.
[55] Borbas C, Morris N, McLaughlin B, et al. The role of clinical opinion leaders in guideline implementation and quality improvement. Chest 2000;118(2 Suppl):24s–32s.
[56] Soumerai SB, Salem-Schatz S, Avorn J, et al. A controlled trial of educational outreach to improve blood transfusion practice. JAMA 1993;270(8):961–6.
[57] Thomson O'Brien MA, Oxman AD, Davis DA, et al. Educational outreach visits: effects on professional practice and health care outcomes. Cochrane Database Syst Rev 2000;(2) Cd000409.
[58] Mazmanian PE, Davis DA. Continuing medical education and the physician as a learner: guide to the evidence. JAMA 2002;288(9):1057–60.
[59] Gorin SS, Ashford AR, Lantigua R, et al. Effectiveness of academic detailing on breast cancer screening among primary care physicians in an underserved community. J Am Board Fam Med 2006;19(2):110–21.
[60] Lobo CM, Frijling BD, Hulscher ME, et al. Improving quality of organizing cardiovascular preventive care in general practice by outreach visitors: a randomized controlled trial. Prev Med 2002;35(5):422–9.
[61] Sinuff T, Cook D, Giacomini M, et al. Facilitating clinician adherence to guidelines in the intensive care unit: a multicenter, qualitative study. Crit Care Med 2007;35(9):2083–9.
[62] Schwann NM, Bretz KA, Eid S, et al. Point-of-care electronic prompts: an effective means of increasing compliance, demonstrating quality, and improving outcome. Anaesth Analg 2011;113(4):869–76.
[63] Jenkins I, Doucet JJ, Clay B, et al. Transfusing wisely: clinical decision support improves blood transfusion practices. Jt Comm J Qual Patient Saf 2017;43(8):389–95.
[64] Ferraris VA, Brown JR, Despotis GJ, et al. 2011 update to the Society of Thoracic Surgeons and the Society of Cardiovascular Anesthesiologists blood conservation clinical practice guidelines. Ann Thorac Surg 2011;91(3):944–82.
[65] Practice guidelines for perioperative blood management: an updated report by the American Society of Anesthesiologists Task Force on Perioperative Blood Management*. Anesthesiology 2015;122(2):241–75.
[66] Kozek-Langenecker SA, Ahmed AB, Afshari A, et al. Management of severe perioperative bleeding: guidelines from the European Society of Anaesthesiology: first update 2016. Eur J Anaesthesiol 2017;34(6):332–95.
[67] Semlitsch T, Blank WA, Kopp IB, et al. Evaluating guidelines: a review of key quality criteria. Dtsch Arztebl Int 2015;112(27–28):471–8.
[68] Coroneos CJ, Voineskos SH, Cornacchi SD, et al. Users' guide to the surgical literature: how to evaluate clinical practice guidelines. Can J Surg 2014;57(4):280–6.

[69] Brouwers MC, Kho ME, Browman GP, et al. The global rating scale complements the AGREE II in advancing the quality of practice guidelines. J Clin Epidemiol 2012;65(5): 526–34.
[70] Siebenhofer A, Semlitsch T, Herborn T, et al. Validation and reliability of a guideline appraisal mini-checklist for daily practice use. BMC Med Res Methodol 2016;16:39.
[71] Grimmer K, Dizon JM, Milanese S, et al. Efficient clinical evaluation of guideline quality: development and testing of a new tool. BMC Med Res Methodol 2014;14:63.
[72] Ferraris VA, Ferraris SP, Saha SP, et al. Perioperative blood transfusion and blood conservation in cardiac surgery: the Society of Thoracic Surgeons and The Society of Cardiovascular Anesthesiologists clinical practice guideline. Ann Thorac Surg 2007;83(5 Suppl): S27–86.
[73] Likosky DS, FitzGerald DC, Groom RC, et al. Effect of the perioperative blood transfusion and blood conservation in cardiac surgery clinical practice guidelines of the Society of Thoracic Surgeons and the Society of Cardiovascular Anesthesiologists upon clinical practices. Anaesth Analg 2010;111(2):316–23.
[74] Woolf SH. Unhealthy medicine, all breathrough, no follow-through. The Washington Post. Available at: https://www.washingtonpost.com/archive/opinions/2006/01/08/unhealthy-medicine-span-classbankheadall-breakthrough-no-follow-throughspan/d3b838a9-db0b-4b23-a410-c5de185f51d0. Accessed August 7, 2019.
[75] Proctor EK, Landsverk J, Aarons G, et al. Implementation research in mental health services: an emerging science with conceptual, methodological, and training challenges. Adm Policy Ment Health 2009;36(1):24–34.
[76] Lobb R, Colditz GA. Implementation science and its application to population health. Annu Rev Public Health 2013;34:235–51.
[77] Handley MA, Gorukanti A, Cattamanchi A. Strategies for implementing implementation science: a methodological overview. Emerg Med J 2016;33(9):660–4.
[78] Michie S. Implementation science: understanding behaviour change and maintenance. BMC Health Serv Res 2014;14(Suppl 2):O9.
[79] Meybohm P, Richards T, Isbister J, et al. Patient blood management bundles to facilitate implementation. Transfus Med Rev 2017;31(1):62–71.
[80] Proctor E, Silmere H, Raghavan R, et al. Outcomes for implementation research: conceptual distinctions, measurement challenges, and research agenda. Adm Policy Ment Health 2011;38(2):65–76.
[81] Greilich PE, Phelps ME, Daniel W. Diffusing innovation and best practice in health care. Anesthesiol Clin 2018;36(1):127–41.
[82] Frank SM, Thakkar RN, Podlasek SJ, et al. Implementing a health system-wide patient blood management program with a clinical community approach. Anesthesiology 2017;127(5):754–64.
[83] Haynes AB, Edmondson L, Lipsitz SR, et al. Mortality trends after a voluntary checklist-based surgical safety collaborative. Ann Surg 2017;266(6):923–9.
[84] Haugen AS, Sevdalis N, Søfteland E. Impact of the world health organization surgical safety checklist on patient safety. Anesthesiology 2019;131(2):420–5.
[85] Journal of implementation science. Available at: http://implementation science.biomedcentral.com. Accessed August 7, 2019.
[86] Annual conference on the science of dissemination and implementation in Health. Available at: https://www.academyhealth.org/events. Accessed August 7, 2019.
[87] UCSF Department of epidemiology and biostatistics. Available at: http://epibiostat.ucsf.edu/certificate-programs. Accessed August 7, 2019.
[88] Shander A, Hofmann A, Ozawa S, et al. The true cost of red blood cell transfusion in surgical patients. Blood 2008;112(11):3045.
[89] Hofmann A, Farmer S, Towler SC. Strategies to preempt and reduce the use of blood products: an Australian perspective. Curr Opin Anaesthesiol 2012;25(1):66–73.

[90] Resar R, Griffin FA, Haraden C, Nolan TW. Using Care Bundles to Improve Health Care Quality. IHI Innovation Series white paper. Cambridge, Massachusetts: Institute for Healthcare Improvement. Available at: http://www.ihi.org. Accessed August 9, 2019.
[91] von Heymann C, Kaufner L, Sander M, et al. Does the severity of preoperative anemia or blood transfusion have a stronger impact on long-term survival after cardiac surgery? J Thorac Cardiovasc Surg 2016;152(5):1412–20.
[92] Bhaskar B, Dulhunty J, Mullany DV, et al. Impact of blood product transfusion on short and long-term survival after cardiac surgery: more evidence. Ann Thorac Surg 2012;94(2):460–7.
[93] Miceli A, Romeo F, Glauber M, et al. Preoperative anemia increases mortality and postoperative morbidity after cardiac surgery. J Cardiothorac Surg 2014;9:137.
[94] Ranucci M, Di Dedda U, Castelvecchio S, et al. Impact of preoperative anemia on outcome in adult cardiac surgery: a propensity-matched analysis. Ann Thorac Surg 2012;94(4):1134–41.
[95] Williams ML, He X, Rankin JS, et al. Preoperative hematocrit is a powerful predictor of adverse outcomes in coronary artery bypass graft surgery: a report from the Society of Thoracic Surgeons Adult Cardiac Surgery Database. Ann Thorac Surg 2013;96(5):1628–34 [discussion: 1634].
[96] Cladellas M, Farre N, Comin-Colet J, et al. Effects of preoperative intravenous erythropoietin plus iron on outcome in anemic patients after cardiac valve replacement. Am J Cardiol 2012;110(7):1021–6.
[97] Yoo YC, Shim JK, Kim JC, et al. Effect of single recombinant human erythropoietin injection on transfusion requirements in preoperatively anemic patients undergoing valvular heart surgery. Anesthesiology 2011;115(5):929–37.
[98] Jimenez K, Kulnigg-Dabsch S, Gasche C. Management of iron deficiency anemia. Gastroenterol Hepatol 2015;11(4):241–50.
[99] Litton E, Xiao J, Ho KM. Safety and efficacy of intravenous iron therapy in reducing requirement for allogeneic blood transfusion: systematic review and meta-analysis of randomised clinical trials. BMJ 2013;347:f4822.
[100] Cho BC, Serini J, Zorrilla-Vaca A, et al. Impact of preoperative erythropoietin on allogeneic blood transfusions in surgical patients: results from a systematic review and meta-analysis. Anaesth Analg 2019;128(5):981–92.
[101] Kei T, Mistry N, Curley G, et al. Efficacy and safety of erythropoietin and iron therapy to reduce red blood cell transfusion in surgical patients: a systematic review and meta-analysis. Can J Anaesth 2019;66(6):716–31.
[102] Weltert L, D'Alessandro S, Nardella S, et al. Preoperative very short-term, high-dose erythropoietin administration diminishes blood transfusion rate in off-pump coronary artery bypass: a randomized blind controlled study. J Thorac Cardiovasc Surg 2010;139(3):621–6 [discussion: 626–7].
[103] Weltert L, Rondinelli B, Bello R, et al. A single dose of erythropoietin reduces perioperative transfusions in cardiac surgery: results of a prospective single-blind randomized controlled trial. Transfusion 2015;55(7):1644–54.
[104] National Collaborating Centre for Chronic Conditions, Royal College of Physicians. Guideline on anaemia management in chronic kidney disease. United Kingdom: National Institute for Clinical Excellence; 2015. Available at: http://www.nice.org.uk/guidance/NG8/evidence. Accessed June 15, 2019.
[105] Locatelli F, Aljama P, Barany P, et al. Revised European best practice guidelines for the management of anaemia in patients with chronic renal failure. Nephrol Dial Transplant 2004;19(Suppl 2):ii1–47.
[106] IV. NKF-K/DOQI clinical practice guidelines for anemia of chronic kidney disease: update 2000. Am J Kidney Dis 2001;37(1 Suppl 1):S182–238.
[107] Nuttall GA, Stehling LC, Beighley CM, et al. Current transfusion practices of members of the American Society of Anesthesiologists: a survey. Anesthesiology 2003;99(6):1433–43.

[108] Stover EP, Siegel LC, Parks R, et al. Variability in transfusion practice for coronary artery bypass surgery persists despite national consensus guidelines: a 24-institution study. Institutions of the Multicenter Study of Perioperative Ischemia Research Group. Anesthesiology 1998;88(2):327–33.
[109] Goodnough LT, Johnston MF, Toy PT. The variability of transfusion practice in coronary artery bypass surgery. Transfusion Medicine Academic Award Group. Jama 1991;265(1): 86–90.
[110] Famolaro T, Yount N, Hare R, et al. Hospital survey on patient safety culture 2018 user database report. (Prepared by Westat, Rockville, MD, under Contract No. HHSA 290201300003C). Rockville (MD): Agency for Healthcare Research and Quality; 2018 AHRQ Publication No. 18-0025-EF.
[111] Anesthesia Quality Institute. 2019 QCDR measure specifications. Version2.1 2019. Available at: https://www.aqihb.org/files/MIPS/2019/2019_QCDR_Measure_Book.pdf. Accessed May 29, 2019.
[112] Story DA, Tait AR. Survey research. Anesthesiology 2019;130(2):192–202.
[113] Lugtenberg M, Burgers JS, Westert GP. Effects of evidence-based clinical practice guidelines on quality of care: a systematic review. Qual Saf Health Care 2009;18(5):385–92.
[114] Freedman J, Luke K, Escobar M, et al. Experience of a network of transfusion coordinators for blood conservation (Ontario Transfusion Coordinators [ONTraC]). Transfusion 2008;48(2):237–50.
[115] Moskowitz DM, McCullough JN, Shander A, et al. The impact of blood conservation on outcomes in cardiac surgery: is it safe and effective? Ann Thorac Surg 2010;90(2):451–8.
[116] Yaffee DW, Smith DE 3rd, Ursomanno PA, et al. Management of blood transfusion in aortic valve surgery: impact of a blood conservation strategy. Ann Thorac Surg 2014;97(1): 95–101.
[117] Gorlinger K, Dirkmann D, Hanke AA. Potential value of transfusion protocols in cardiac surgery. Curr Opin Anaesthesiol 2013;26(2):230–43.
[118] Nuttall GA, Oliver WC, Santrach PJ, et al. Efficacy of a simple intraoperative transfusion algorithm for nonerythrocyte component utilization after cardiopulmonary bypass. Anesthesiology 2001;94(5):773–81 [discussion: 775A–6A].
[119] LaPar DJ, Crosby IK, Ailawadi G, et al. Blood product conservation is associated with improved outcomes and reduced costs after cardiac surgery. J Thorac Cardiovasc Surg 2013;145(3):796–803 [discussion: 803–4].
[120] Pearse BL, Smith I, Faulke D, et al. Protocol guided bleeding management improves cardiac surgery patient outcomes. Vox Sang 2015;109(3):267–79.
[121] Karkouti K, Callum J, Wijeysundera DN, et al. Point-of-care hemostatic testing in cardiac surgery: a stepped-wedge clustered randomized controlled trial. Circulation 2016;134(16):1152–62.
[122] Weber CF, Gorlinger K, Meininger D, et al. Point-of-care testing: a prospective, randomized clinical trial of efficacy in coagulopathic cardiac surgery patients. Anesthesiology 2012;117(3):531–47.
[123] Shore-Lesserson L, Manspeizer HE, DePerio M, et al. Thromboelastography-guided transfusion algorithm reduces transfusions in complex cardiac surgery. Anesth Analg 1999;88(2):312–9.
[124] Mazer CD, Whitlock RP, Fergusson DA, et al. Six-month outcomes after restrictive or liberal transfusion for cardiac surgery. N Engl J Med 2018;379(13):1224–33.
[125] Xydas S, Magovern CJ, Slater JP, et al. Implementation of a comprehensive blood conservation program can reduce blood use in a community cardiac surgery program. J Thorac Cardiovasc Surg 2012;143(4):926–35.
[126] Ternstrom L, Hyllner M, Backlund E, et al. A structured blood conservation programme reduces transfusions and costs in cardiac surgery. Interact Cardiovasc Thorac Surg 2014;19(5):788–94.

[127] Chu MW, Losenno KL, Moore K, et al. Blood conservation strategies reduce the need for transfusions in ascending and aortic arch surgery. Perfusion 2013;28(4):315–21.
[128] Fleisher LA, Fleischmann KE, Auerbach AD, et al. 2014 ACC/AHA guideline on perioperative cardiovascular evaluation and management of patients undergoing noncardiac surgery: a report of the American College of Cardiology/American Heart Association Task Force on practice guidelines. J Am Coll Cardiol 2014;64(22):e77–137.
[129] Carson JL, Grossman BJ, Kleinman S, et al. Red blood cell transfusion: a clinical practice guideline from the AABB*. Ann Intern Med 2012;157(1):49–58.

APPENDIX 1: STANDARDS FOR DEVELOPING TRUSTWORTHY CLINICAL PRACTICE GUIDELINES

STANDARD 1

Establishing transparency

1.1 The processes by which a CPG is developed and funded should be detailed explicitly and publicly accessible.

STANDARD 2

Management of conflict of interest (COI)

2.1 Prior to selection of the Guideline Development Group (GDG), individuals being considered for membership should declare all interests and activities potentially resulting in COI with development group activity, by written disclosure to those convening the GDG.
- Disclosure should reflect all current and planned commercial (including services from which a clinician derives a substantial proportion of income), noncommercial, intellectual, institutional, and patient/public activities pertinent to the potential scope of the CPG.

2.2 Disclosure of COIs within GDG
- All COI of each GDG member should be reported and discussed by the prospective development group prior to the onset of their work.
- Each panel member should explain how their COI could influence the CPG development process or specific recommendations.

2.3 Divestment
- Members of the GDG should divest themselves of financial investments they or their family members have in, and not participate in marketing activities or advisory boards of, entities whose interests could be affected by CPG recommendations.

2.4 Exclusions
- Whenever possible GDG members should not have COI.
- In some circumstances, a GDG may not be able to perform its work without members who have COIs, such as relevant clinical specialists who receive a substantial portion of their incomes from services pertinent to the CPG.
- Members with COIs should represent not more than a minority of the GDG.
- The chair or co-chairs should not be a person(s) with COI.
- Funders should have no role in CPG development.

CLINICAL DESCRIPTION

The clinical presentation of MH can vary. It can be difficult to diagnose MH with confidence in the absence of diagnostic testing, especially while the patient is receiving general anesthesia [12]. All halogenated inhalational anesthetic agents currently in use (isoflurane, sevoflurane, desflurane) are potential triggering agents for MH. Succinylcholine, a depolarizing neuromuscular relaxant, is also a known triggering agent. Studies in pigs validate succinylcholine as a trigger, and it is known that succinylcholine can potentiate the MH reaction from volatile anesthetics [13]. No other anesthetic agents, including nitrous oxide, currently in use have been identified as potential triggering agents [2].

MH most often occurs intraoperatively with exposure to triggering agents. It can present in the early postoperative period, but in most cases review of the anesthetic record reveals that diagnostic clues were present sooner. Because MH is a muscle-based hypermetabolic process, the hallmark of MH is increased carbon dioxide production. When a patient's ventilation is being controlled, the clinician has to adjust ventilator parameters to compensate for elimination of this additional carbon dioxide, which should be an early indication of a potential MH crisis. In cases in which a patient is breathing spontaneously, increased minute ventilation may go unnoticed until the production of carbon dioxide exceeds the patient's ability to compensate, contributing to delay in diagnosis [14].

Another early sign of MH is unexplained sinus tachycardia. Because sinus tachycardia is a common and nonspecific sign, it may be misdiagnosed as being caused by a light plane of anesthesia or inadequate pain control. Tachycardia combined with hypercarbia is highly suspicious of a hypermetabolic state, and an evaluation to confirm or exclude MH should be ruled out by assessing the patient for muscle rigidity, acidosis, or hyperkalemia [15].

Hyperthermia is a key indicator of MH, but it can be a late sign or may be absent [16]. However, rapidly increasing core temperature is more commonly noted if hypermetabolism is present for any significant period of time. Delay in diagnosis and hyperthermia greater than 39°C has been shown to increase the risk of morbidity from organ dysfunction/failure and from DIC. Isolated temperature increases at any point, unaccompanied by associated signs of hypermetabolism (hypercarbia/tachycardia), are unlikely to be MH [17]. Skin liquid crystal temperature indicators have failed in numerous reports and their use should be discouraged in favor of more reliable patient temperature monitoring.

Generalized muscle rigidity is seen in 50% to 80% of patients, caused by muscle contraction, and is an important and highly specific sign of MH [1]. Rhabdomyolysis, breakdown of skeletal muscle, is a late sign of MH and can result in life-threatening hyperkalemia. Myoglobinuria from rhabdomyolysis may also lead to acute renal failure [18].

Other clinical signs of MH may include hypoxemia, pulmonary edema, congestive heart failure, cardiac arrhythmias, electrolyte imbalances, and alterations in consciousness [3].

Medical conditions such as sepsis, pheochromocytoma, neuroleptic malignant syndrome, serotonin syndrome, and thyroid storm may resemble the pattern of MH and may be difficult to differentiate on clinical basis alone [8].

Treatment algorithim

If feasible, end surgery as soon as possible, and stop all triggering agents.

If surgery must proceed, begin nontriggering anesthetic with IV agents.

Call for help, and obtain dantrolene and MH supplies. Call emergency services if transfer to tertiary facility is required for intensive care unit (ICU)–level care. Call the Malignant Hyperthermia Association of the United States (MHAUS) Hotline for assistance 24/7 (1-800-644-9737).

Hyperventilate and use high flows of oxygen at fraction of inspired oxygen 1.0 to flush volatile anesthetics from the breathing circuit and to help quickly decrease end-tidal CO2 (ETCO2). Use inline charcoal filters, if available, to quickly scrub trace gases from the circuit.

As soon as possible, administer dantrolene 2.5 mg/kg IV. If using standard dantrolene, mix the drug using 60 mL of sterile water. Several assistants may be necessary. Administer each vial as soon as reconstituted until the loading dose is complete. Additional dantrolene may be given up to 10 mg/kg as needed to decrease ETCO2, stabilize vital signs, or end rigidity. Ryanodex (lyophilized preparation of dantrolene) requires 5 mL of sterile water per 250 mg.

Laboratories should include arterial blood gas (ABG), serum potassium, and creatine kinase (CK) levels, along with urine myoglobin level. Follow ABGs for resolution of acidosis. Repeat CK measurements every 6 hours until returned to normal in order to diagnose and treat possible rhabdomyolysis.

Actively cool the patient if core temperature is increased. Stop cooling when the temperature has decreased to less than 38_C, to avoid hypothermia. Patients can be cooled with ambient air; ice packs to groin, axilla, and head; intraperitoneal lavage; or Cardiopulmonary Bypass.

Treat hyperkalemia with calcium, glucose, and insulin, as well as bicarbonate as necessary.

Avoid calcium channel blockers in the treatment of arrhythmias, because they can precipitate hyperkalemia and cardiac collapse.

Give IV fluids/diuretics to ensure greater than 1 mL/kg/h urine output. Dantrolene has small amount of mannitol added as a buffering agent; more may be required if rhabdomyolysis present. Treat acidosis and hyperkalemia if present (discussed earlier).

If CK or Kþ level increases, assume myoglobinuria is present and give bicarbonate infusion of 1 mEq/kg/h, to alkalinize urine.

Continue to monitor urine output, core temperature, ETCO2, and pH as indicated. Arrange for transport to a critical care setting as symptoms resolve.

TREATMENT

The antidote drug, dantrolene, was approved by the US Food and Drug Administration in 1979 for use in MH crisis. It is a muscle relaxant drug that acts as an antagonist at the ryanodine receptor to slow the release of calcium and to allow the cells to reincorporate it into the sarcoplasmic reticulum. Given as a loading dose of 2.5 mg/kg IV, it rapidly slows the hypermetabolic process involved in MH. There are 2 commonly dispensed preparations. The standard preparation is Dantrium, available in 20-mg vials that require 60 mL of sterile water to reconstitute. Giving a 2.5-mg/kg loading dose to the average 100-kg patient requires multiple providers to proceed efficiently. A newer, more concentrated preparation is Ryanodex, supplied in vials containing 250 mg of dantrolene requiring only 5 mL of sterile water to reconstitute. Some clinicians question the cost-effectiveness of routinely stocking dantrolene, given the low incidence of MH, the cost of the drug (higher with the Ryanodex), and the limited (3-year) shelf life. A recent review [19] confirms dantrolene's cost-effectiveness compared with supportive care alone in the outpatient setting. MHAUS strongly recommends stocking dantrolene at any facility in which triggering agents are being used.

Before dantrolene use became widely popular in the early 1980s, only 36% of patients survived when treatment was limited to the symptoms of MH [20]. Modern MH mortality in patients less than 18 years old ranges from 0.66% to 4.6% [20–23]. A significantly lower mortality is reliably shown in children versus adults, possibly secondary to earlier diagnosis and treatment. According to National Inpatient Sample (NIS) data, mortality for adults (14.1%) was significantly higher than in pediatric patients (0.7%). Mortality did significantly increase as the number of comorbidities increased in the adult and pediatric populations [24]. The significantly better mortality seen in pediatric versus adult patients is directly attributable to early recognition and treatment with dantrolene. Another explanation for the improved mortality is the decreased use of succinylcholine in the pediatric population [24]. Statistically significant higher mortality has been observed among pediatric patients in the southern United States, those with higher comorbidities, in patients transferred between facilities, or those listed as having been admitted through the emergency department [24]. In addition, an alarming complication rate (35%) still exists for MH-treated patients [6]. Studies have shown that complication rates and morbidity increase with a muscular build, with increased time between induction and highest $ETCO_2$, and with development of DIC. Only 6.5% of patients had a prior family history of MH [20].

An attempt should be to collect blood for laboratory electrolyte and CK analysis before dantrolene is given, to assist in confirming the diagnosis. Clinicians should be cautious with extreme cooling measures in children because the cutaneous vasoconstriction seen with intense cooling may reduce the ability to discharge heat and reduce skeletal blood flow, contributing to worse patient outcomes. Despite decreases in MH-related mortality and improved MH recognition in recent decades, fatal MH cases still occur because of the variable presentation, lack of dantrolene availability or administration, and inappropriate or incomplete treatment [25].

Dantrolene is well tolerated clinically, although side effects do occur in up to 21.6% of treated patients. The most commonly described side effect is muscle weakness, and patients treated with high doses of dantrolene may require ventilator support. Phlebitis, rash, and transaminitis have also been described [22].

RECRUDESCENCE

Recrudescence is the recurrence of MH symptoms following successful initial treatment. In one study, recrudescence occurred in 14.4% of patients less than 18 years old and in 19.1% of children less than 12 years old [22]. A second study found the recrudescence rate to be 20% for all pediatric patients, and slightly higher at 29% for children less than 12 years old [26]. Two cases were fatal: one occurred in a 4-year-old 6 hours after initial MH symptoms resolved, and the second case was in a 14-year-old in whom symptoms recurred 24 hours after initial symptom resolution [22]. The North American MH Registry (NAMHR) database found the mean onset time for recrudescence to be 13 hours in 308 pediatric patients; 73% of these patients were male. Further analysis showed that recrudescence was more likely with a muscular body type, Clinical Grading Scale (CGS) score greater than 35, greater than 150 minutes from induction to peak symptoms, or presence of a temperature increase noted with initial symptoms [27].

It is critical for anesthesiologists to consider recrudescence following initial treatment and to take an active role in managing the ICU courses of patients with MH. The risk of recrudescence increases with greater muscle mass, and can occur at times remote from initial treatment and apparent recovery [26].

EPIDEMIOLOGY

A clear understanding of MH has been challenged by the dominant reliance on case reports and retrospective studies. It is not possible to perform prospective randomized human trials because of the ethical concern of exposing susceptible patients to a known trigger. Understanding MH risk factors, prevalence, and outcomes requires very large databases to account for the rarity of the disease and the variability in its presentation [21].

Multiple databases exist and have been used to analyze data regarding MH, including the NAMHR, which was established in 1987 and merged with the MHAUS in 1995 so that data on MH could be stored in a single site. In addition, the Kids' Inpatient Database (KID) is the largest publicly available all-payer pediatric inpatient care database in the United States, containing information from approximately 3 million pediatric discharges each year. The KID has been produced every 3 years from 1997 to 2016. Pediatric data have also been extracted from the NIS, which is another publicly available all-payer inpatient health care database in the United States that includes pediatric hospital inpatient stays not including outpatient surgery. Extremely large databases such as these have been successfully used to analyze MH data. The International Classification of Disease, Ninth Version (ICD-9), code for MH (995.86) was introduced in 1998. However, there are inherent risks and missed patients with retrospective database reviews that have been based on ICD-9 coding. Despite MH having a unique ICD-9 code, it is probable that some patients were either misdiagnosed or miscoded.

INCIDENCE/MORTALITY

The exact clinical incidence of MH is unknown, but it is estimated that MH occurs in 1 in 15,000 children and 1 in 50,000 adults undergoing an anesthetic [5]. The incidence reported in the literature varies widely; from 1:14,000 anesthetics put forth by Britt [5] to the values reported by Rosero and colleagues [24] of 1 to 1.3 per 100,000, or by Li and colleagues [23] at 3 per 100,000. The 13 years of data reviewed by Salazar and colleagues [21], using NIS and KID data, revealed an incidence of 0.1 per 100,000, whereas Brady and colleagues [28] analyzed New York State date over a 5-year period and reported an incidence of 1 per 100,000, but found the MH risk significantly higher in men than in women. New York State inpatient data from 2001 to 2005 showed a consistent MH incidence among pediatric patients less than 18 years old. The MH rate was 1 in 100,000 for surgical anesthetics, and 4.4 in 100,000 for nonsurgical anesthetic cases [28].

Prevalence analyzed by age shows that children between the age of 1 and 4 years had an increased prevalence of 5.6 in 100,000 compared with all pediatric patients. Boys were 3 times more likely at 4.9 versus 1.6 in 100,000 for girls ($P < .00001$), but the sex difference for MH prevalence was not seen in infants. In addition, no differences were seen in pediatric MH prevalence with regard to race, year of admission, and admission type; that is, scheduled versus unscheduled [23]. Of note, cases of MH among pediatric patients were approximately equally split between pediatric hospitals and nonpediatric hospitals [21].

The prevalence of genetic variants or mutations that make an individual MH susceptible is estimated to be between 1 in 2000 and 1 in 3000, which is notably discrepant and higher than the incidence of clinical MH [29]. MH is thought to follow an autosomal dominant pattern of inheritance with incomplete penetrance and variable expression [30–33]. Incomplete penetrance of a genetic trait means that the phenotype may not be expressed in every individual that carries the allele, and that it may require additional factors for expression of the disease phenotype. This finding may be caused by multiple genes operating together or against each other to express a certain phenotype. Variable expression means that individuals carrying the same allele may display different phenotypes. There is evidence for the presence of genetic factors influencing penetrance and expression, but specific factors are poorly understood. Incomplete penetrance and variable expression make the disorder even harder to characterize [34,35]. The discrepancy between the clinical incidence of MH and the prevalence of genetic susceptibility variants may be explained by these complex patterns of inheritance and expression [29].

MH may develop when a susceptible individual is exposed to a trigger for the first time; however, susceptible patients on average undergo 3 anesthetics

mapping the genetic information for a host of myopathic conditions that before now were associated with MH via rare case reports. The overarching theme is that myopathies genuinely associated with MH almost invariably are in individuals with RYR1 gain-of-function mutations, or, more infrequently, CACNA1S. Gain-of-function mutations are those that shift systems toward threshold levels. The disorders most likely directly linked are central core disease (CCD) and King-Denborough syndrome. CCD is often diagnosed in early infancy with generalized weakness and skeletal deformities. Affected infants show dominantly inherited RYR1 variants with MH phenotype. Second, King-Denborough syndrome is extremely rare and is associated with dysmorphic features and skeletal anomalies, including kyphoscoliosis, pectus carinatum, and short stature, and myopathy [25,49–51]. They too show RYR1 mutations with MH phenotype [52].

The most commonly reported associated diagnosis in pediatric MH cases is rhabdomyolysis, which occurred in 26% of the cases in the KID and NIS datasets. Muscular dystrophy and mitochondrial disorders were the most common comorbidity, but most often do not truly represent MH. Dystrophic muscle (Duchenne and Becker muscular dystrophy) can show rhabdomyolysis and brief rigidity on exposure to inhalational anesthetics and catastrophic hyperkalemia from rhabdomyolysis following succinylcholine administration, but that is not MH [52].

Hypotonia is a common diagnosis in children and presents a unique challenge to anesthesiologists. Most hypotonia in children is either central in origin (central nervous system dysfunction secondary to chronic hypoxic ischemic encephalopathy) or secondary to chromosomal abnormalities such as trisomy 21. Hypotonia in pediatric patients does not increase MH susceptibility, and a nontriggering anesthetic is not necessary [52]. Younger patients were more likely to show muscle weakness, undescended testes, and inguinal hernia [22].

Case reports of confirmed MH episodes in the absence of triggering agents have led some investigators to search for a link between MH, exertional rhabdomyolysis (ER), and exertional heat illness (EHI) [53,54]. The conditions share many clinical similarities, including increased core temperatures, muscle rigidity, tachycardia, tachypnea, increased CK level, hyperkalemia, myoglobinuria, acute renal failure, and DIC. Dantrolene has proved an effective treatment in cases of EHI. Interestingly, cohort studies have shown MH-associated RYR1 mutations in up to 30% of patients with ER studied [54]. However, when MH pedigree families are queried, even those with mutations known to be highly pathogenic, no increased rates of ER or EHI are found. Further, when patients with a history of either ER or EHI are studied, most mutations found are variants of unknown significance [30]. Patients with history of ER/EHI and RYR1 mutations may simply have overlapping but causally unlinked diagnoses. Further investigation is warranted, and patients with ER/EHI should have detailed genetic analysis looking for RYR1 and CACNA1S mutations, along with screening for myopathy/rhabdomyolysis disorders.

Children often show a heterogeneous presentation of MH, and their diagnosis can be delayed [55]. In 1994, Larach and colleagues [56] developed a CGS for MH recognition using clinical indicators to predict the likelihood of an MH event. The following 6 indicators were identified: (1) muscle rigidity, (2) muscle breakdown (increased CK level or myoglobinuria), (3) respiratory acidosis or hypercarbia, (4) temperature increase (single hyperthermic episode or a rapid increase in temperature), (5) cardiac involvement (tachyarrhythmia or ventricular arrhythmia), and (6) family history of MH. The raw score from all 6 indicators is tallied from 0 to 50+, and an MH rank from 0 to 6 is totaled (6 being the most likely). In addition, a description of the likelihood of an MH reaction is assigned a phrase with a range from "almost never" to "almost certain." The CGS for MH is a very valuable tool to assist in early MH recognition and is often used in retrospective reviews to confirm the diagnosis. Organizations such as the MHAUS use a similar grading scale when anesthesiologists phone the hotline to discuss a case and decide the likelihood of MH and whether to treat. Because most pediatric presentations are not classic presentations, it is extremely helpful to use the CGS to assist in diagnosis [25].

Historically, temporomandibular joint or masseter spasm occurred in 1% of mask inductions with halothane and succinylcholine. However, these reactions were self-limited and dantrolene was rarely given. Masseter spasm is rarely seen now that halothane and succinylcholine are used less frequently [57]. Often case reports and older studies routinely included masseter spasm as an early clue to an MH reaction, but modern anesthetics do not routinely use either agent so anesthesiologists must be aware of other presenting signs.

In a study done by Nelson and Litman [22] in 2014, using NAMHR data, 351 subjects from 1960 to 2011 were reviewed for MH using the CGS scale and 264 or 75.2% of patients met the criteria for almost-certain MH. The patients were then separated into 3 categories to better define any possible presentation trends among the pediatric population. Thirty-five children were in the youngest (0–24 months) age group, 163 were in the middle (25 months to 12 years) age group, and 66 were in the oldest (13–18 years) age group. The likelihood of the condition being seen in male patients increased with age, and was most pronounced in the oldest group. A family history of MH was present in 18.5% of patients with MH. The MH event occurred with the first anesthetic in 50% of patients and during the second anesthetic in 20% of patients. The investigators hypothesized that earlier recognition of MH might occur if more common presentations per pediatric age group could be identified. Across the entire pediatric range, sinus tachycardia was the first sign of an MH crisis in 73.1% of cases, hypercarbia was seen second in 68.6%, and a rapid temperature increase was seen in 48.5%. The oldest group of patients were most likely to develop all 3 and to reach the highest maximum temperature. It is thus helpful to understand that teenaged patients are more likely to develop classic MH symptoms of tachycardia, hypercarbia, and hyperthermia. The greater muscle mass typically present may explain the more common classic presentation of MH that is seen in older children. This possibility is further supported by the fact that teenaged patients develop higher peak CK and potassium levels, and a greater degree of rhabdomyolysis, when they have MH. Patients aged 2 to 12 years more typically developed lower peak $ETCO_2$and $PaCO_2$ but were more likely to show masseter spasm, especially if succinylcholine was used. This middle group (2–12 years) was the most heterogeneous group with regard to presentation. The youngest patients (<2 years) more frequently showed skin mottling, were half as likely to show muscle rigidity, and developed higher peak lactic acid and lower peak CK levels, likely secondary to higher resting metabolic rates and decreased muscle reserve. This study by Nelson and Litman [22] highlights the variety of MH symptoms that can be seen in pediatric MH crisis.

SPECIAL SCENARIOS/DIFFERENTIAL DIAGNOSIS

Despite earlier recognition and better survival among the pediatric population, there are a few special circumstances that any anesthesiologist that cares for children should consider. Brandom and Muldoon [58] in 2013 described multiple fatal pediatric MH cases without exposure to triggering agents. Common elements seen were muscle rigidity; increased temperature; cardiovascular collapse; and, on follow-up review, an abnormal RYR type 1 gene. Some patients with MH without a triggering exposure had a recent viral illness, but that was not uniformly seen. As discussed earlier, the presentation of MH is highly variable in children, and a wide differential diagnosis must be considered even if a nontriggering anesthetic is used. Anesthesia-induced rhabdomyolysis (AIR) should be considered early in the setting of a patient being considered for MH. Both AIR and MH have similar presentations with hyperthermia and muscle rigidity, but the early treatment strategies are different. AIR should be more strongly considered in any patient with a known history of muscle myopathies. Essential treatment of AIR is calcium and cardiovascular support, whereas IV dantrolene is critical in the treatment of MH.

An additional consideration in the future of MH treatment involves earlier recognition of MH with advanced electronic detection and clinical decision support. A group at Mayo Clinic has developed and tested an electronic medical record (EMR) MH detection tool, which they have applied to 10 years of data. Their EMR tool was used to analyze data in a model of the flow in an operating room. The real-time detection device or "data sniffer" was reported to be sufficiently sensitive that providers would have been alerted earlier than recognition occurred during the original event [59]. It is a novel approach to MH recognition and treatment that will be explored further in the future.

SUMMARY

MH remains a relevant clinical emergency in anesthesia more than 50 years after its characterization, and 40 years after the development of the antidote drug, dantrolene. Advances in genetic testing and research have yielded vast amounts of information about the electrochemical processes involved and the genetic mutations responsible for MH events, but contracture testing continues to be a key element in establishing phenotype. The shared goal is vigilance in monitoring and efficiency in treatment that brings mortality from MH to zero.

References

[1] Kim DC. Malignant hyperthermia. Korean J Anesthesiol 2012;63(5):391–401.
[2] Hopkins PM. Malignant hyperthermia: pharmacology of triggering. Br J Anaesth 2011;107(1):48–56.
[3] Rosenberg H, et al. Malignant hyperthermia: a review. Orphanet J Rare Dis 2015;10:93.
[4] Lopez JR, et al. Malignant hyperthermia, environmental heat stress, and intracellular calcium dysregulation in a mouse model expressing the p.G2435R variant of RYR1. Br J Anaesth 2018;121(4):953–61.
[5] Britt BA, Kalow W. Malignant hyperthermia: a statistical review. Can Anaesth Soc J 1970;17(4):293–315.
[6] Larach MG, et al. Clinical presentation, treatment, and complications of malignant hyperthermia in North America from 1987 to 2006. Anesth Analg 2010;110(2):498–507.
[7] Larach MG, et al. Malignant hyperthermia deaths related to inadequate temperature monitoring, 2007-2012: a report from the North American malignant hyperthermia registry of the malignant hyperthermia association of the United States. Anesth Analg 2014;119(6): 1359–66.
[8] Rosenberg H, et al. Malignant hyperthermia. Orphanet J Rare Dis 2007;2:21.
[9] Nelson TE, Sweo T. Ca2+ uptake and Ca2+ release by skeletal muscle sarcoplasmic reticulum: differing sensitivity to inhalational anesthetics. Anesthesiology 1988;69(4):571–7.
[10] Iaizzo PA, Klein W, Lehmann-Horn F. Fura-2 detected myoplasmic calcium and its correlation with contracture force in skeletal muscle from normal and malignant hyperthermia susceptible pigs. Pflugers Arch 1988;411(6):648–53.
[11] Yang T, et al. Enhanced excitation-coupled calcium entry in myotubes is associated with expression of RyR1 malignant hyperthermia mutations. J Biol Chem 2007;282(52): 37471–8.
[12] Hopkins PM. Malignant hyperthermia: advances in clinical management and diagnosis. Br J Anaesth 2000;85(1):118–28.
[13] Schuster F, et al. BMC Anesthesiol 2014;14:14.
[14] Karan SM, Crowl F, Muldoon SM. Malignant hyperthermia masked by capnographic monitoring. Anesth Analg 1994;78(3):590–2.
[15] Romanovsky AA. Thermoregulation: from basic neuroscience to clinical neurology; part II 2018.
[16] Ali SZ, Taguchi A, Rosenberg H. Malignant hyperthermia. Best Pract Res Clin Anaesthesiol 2003;17(4):519–33.
[17] Nelson TE. Porcine malignant hyperthermia: critical temperatures for in vivo and in vitro responses. Anesthesiology 1990;73(3):449–54.
[18] McKenney KA, Holman SJ. Delayed postoperative rhabdomyolysis in a patient subsequently diagnosed as malignant hyperthermia susceptible. Anesthesiology 2002;96(3): 764–5.
[19] Aderibigbe T, Lang BH, Rosenberg H, et al. Cost-effectiveness analysis of stocking dantrolene in ambulatory surgery centers for the treatment of malignant hyperthermia. Anesthesiology 2014;120:1333–8.
[20] Larach MG, et al. Cardiac arrests and deaths associated with malignant hyperthermia in north america from 1987 to 2006: a report from the north american malignant hyperthermia registry of the malignant hyperthermia association of the United States. Anesthesiology 2008;108(4):603–11.

[21] Salazar JH, et al. Pediatric malignant hyperthermia: risk factors, morbidity, and mortality identified from the Nationwide Inpatient Sample and Kids' Inpatient Database. Paediatr Anaesth 2014;24(12):1212–6.
[22] Nelson P, Litman RS. Malignant hyperthermia in children: an analysis of the North American malignant hyperthermia registry. Anesth Analg 2014;118(2):369–74.
[23] Li G, et al. Excess comorbidities associated with malignant hyperthermia diagnosis in pediatric hospital discharge records. Paediatr Anaesth 2011;21(9):958–63.
[24] Rosero EB, et al. Trends and outcomes of malignant hyperthermia in the United States, 2000 to 2005. Anesthesiology 2009;110(1):89–94.
[25] Lerman J. Perioperative management of the paediatric patient with coexisting neuromuscular disease. Br J Anaesth 2011;107(Suppl 1):i79–89.
[26] Burkman JM, Posner KL, Domino KB. Analysis of the clinical variables associated with recrudescence after malignant hyperthermia reactions. Anesthesiology 2007;106(5):901–6 [quiz: 1077–8].
[27] Lu Z, et al. Prevalence of malignant hyperthermia diagnosis in New York State ambulatory surgery center discharge records 2002 to 2011. Anesth Analg 2016;122(2):449–53.
[28] Brady JE, et al. Prevalence of malignant hyperthermia due to anesthesia in New York State, 2001-2005. Anesth Analg 2009;109(4):1162–6.
[29] Riazi S, Kraeva N, Hopkins PM. Malignant hyperthermia in the post-genomics era: new perspectives on an old concept. Anesthesiology 2018;128(1):168–80.
[30] Fiszer D, et al. Next-generation sequencing of RYR1 and CACNA1S in malignant hyperthermia and exertional heat illness. Anesthesiology 2015;122(5):1033–46.
[31] King JO, Denborough MA, Zapf PW. Inheritance of malignant hyperpyrexia. Lancet 1972;1(7746):365–70.
[32] Monnier N, et al. Presence of two different genetic traits in malignant hyperthermia families: implication for genetic analysis, diagnosis, and incidence of malignant hyperthermia susceptibility. Anesthesiology 2002;97(5):1067–74.
[33] Denborough MA, et al. Anaesthetic deaths in a family. Br J Anaesth 1962;34:395–6.
[34] McCarthy TV, Quane KA, Lynch PJ. Ryanodine receptor mutations in malignant hyperthermia and central core disease. Hum Mutat 2000;15(5):410–7.
[35] Robinson RL, Curran JL, Ellis FR, et al. Multiple interacting gene products may influence susceptibility to malignant hyperthermia. Ann Hum Genet 2000;64:307–20.
[36] MacLennan DH, et al. Ryanodine receptor gene is a candidate for predisposition to malignant hyperthermia. Nature 1990;343(6258):559–61.
[37] Carpenter D, et al. The role of CACNA1S in predisposition to malignant hyperthermia. BMC Med Genet 2009;10:104.
[38] Kim JH, et al. Exome sequencing reveals novel rare variants in the ryanodine receptor and calcium channel genes in malignant hyperthermia families. Anesthesiology 2013;119(5): 1054–65.
[39] Toppin PJ, et al. A report of fulminant malignant hyperthermia in a patient with a novel mutation of the CACNA1S gene. Can J Anaesth 2010;57(7):689–93.
[40] Horstick EJ, et al. Stac3 is a component of the excitation-contraction coupling machinery and mutated in Native American myopathy. Nat Commun 2013;4:1952.
[41] Miller DM, et al. Genetic epidemiology of malignant hyperthermia in the UK. Br J Anaesth 2018;121(4):944–52.
[42] Robinson R, et al. Mutations in RYR1 in malignant hyperthermia and central core disease. Hum Mutat 2006;27(10):977–89.
[43] Sambuughin N, et al. Screening of the entire ryanodine receptor type 1 coding region for sequence variants associated with malignant hyperthermia susceptibility in the north american population. Anesthesiology 2005;102(3):515–21.
[44] Dainese M, et al. Anesthetic- and heat-induced sudden death in calsequestrin-1-knockout mice. FASEB J 2009;23(6):1710–20.

[45] Protasi F, Paolini C, Dainese M. Calsequestrin-1: a new candidate gene for malignant hyperthermia and exertional/environmental heat stroke. J Physiol 2009;587(Pt 13):3095–100.
[46] Kraeva N, et al. CASQ1 gene is an unlikely candidate for malignant hyperthermia susceptibility in the North American population. Anesthesiology 2013;118(2):344–9.
[47] Hopkins PM, et al. genetic epidemiology of the UK malignant hyperthermia cohort. Br J Anaesth 2016;116:937–8.
[48] Allen GC, Larach MG, Kunselman AR. The sensitivity and specificity of the caffeine-halothane contracture test: a report from the North American Malignant Hyperthermia Registry. The North American Malignant Hyperthermia Registry of MHAUS. Anesthesiology 1998;88(3):579–88.
[49] Baraka AS, Jalbout MI. Anesthesia and myopathy. Curr Opin Anaesthesiol 2002;15(3): 371–6.
[50] Benca J, Hogan K. Malignant hyperthermia, coexisting disorders, and enzymopathies: risks and management options. Anesth Analg 2009;109(4):1049–53.
[51] Klingler W, et al. Core myopathies and risk of malignant hyperthermia. Anesth Analg 2009;109(4):1167–73.
[52] Litman RS, et al. Malignant hyperthermia susceptibility and related diseases. Anesthesiology 2018;128(1):159–67.
[53] Timmins MA, et al. Malignant hyperthermia testing in probands without adverse anesthetic reaction. Anesthesiology 2015;123(3):548–56.
[54] Wappler F, et al. Evidence for susceptibility to malignant hyperthermia in patients with exercise-induced rhabdomyolysis. Anesthesiology 2001;94(1):95–100.
[55] Broman M, Islander G, Muller CR. Malignant hyperthermia, a Scandinavian update. Acta Anaesthesiol Scand 2015;59(8):951–61.
[56] Larach MG, et al. A clinical grading scale to predict malignant hyperthermia susceptibility. Anesthesiology 1994;80(4):771–9.
[57] Lazzell VA, et al. The incidence of masseter muscle rigidity after succinylcholine in infants and children. Can J Anaesth 1994;41(6):475–9.
[58] Brandom BW, Muldoon SM. Unexpected MH deaths without exposure to inhalation anesthetics in pediatric patients. Paediatr Anaesth 2013;23(9):851–4.
[59] Gleich SJ, et al. An automated real-time method for the detection of patients at risk for malignant hyperthermia. Paediatr Anaesth 2016;26(9):876–82.

Advances in Anesthesia 37 (2019) 53–63

ADVANCES IN ANESTHESIA

ELSEVIER
MOSBY

History, Current State, and Future of Diversity in the Anesthesia Workforce

Melissa R. Kenevan, MD, Bhargavi Gali, MD*

Department of Anesthesiology and Perioperative Medicine, Mayo Clinic, 200 First Street Southwest, Rochester, MN 55905, USA

Keywords

• Diversity • Health care disparities • Medical faculty • Leadership

Key points

- A diverse workforce, including leadership, has been recognized as an important factor in innovation and economic productivity in the business sector. Companies with higher diversity outperform those with limited diversity.
- As the population increases in diversity, the ability to transform the medical workforce to better care for all patients, in addition to continuing to innovate, depends on the ability to attract more diverse physicians.
- Anesthesia, along with most other medical specialties, lags in attracting diverse physicians. Current efforts, including programs recently developed in neuroanesthesia and the American Society of Anesthesiologists Professional Diversity Committee, are steps toward change.

INTRODUCTION

Diversity is "the condition of having or being composed of differing elements" (Merriam-Webster Dictionary). Taking this a step further, human diversity can be described as inherent, the traits people were born with, or acquired, referring to the traits that are gained from experience [1]. According to the US Census Bureau, the population demographics of the United States are growing more and more diverse. It is estimated that in 2020 more than 50% of the nation's children will be considered of racial and/or ethnic minorities, and in 2044 the United States

Disclosure: The authors have nothing to disclose.

*Corresponding author. *E-mail address:* Gali.Bhargavi@mayo.edu
twitter: @KenevanMelissa (M.R.K.); @bxgali (B.G.)

https://doi.org/10.1016/j.aan.2019.08.001
0737-6146/19/

will become a so-called majority minority nation, with most Americans belonging to a minority group [2]. As this trend continues, many companies and other groups are identifying the importance of organizational inclusion; diversity not only as a matter of social justice but also as a leading factor for enhanced performance and global competitiveness. In medicine, women and minorities have historically been underrepresented in the workforce and this currently holds true in anesthesiology [3]. This article reviews workforce and leadership diversity in medicine, and more specifically in anesthesiology, and its implications for health care disparities and the future of this specialty.

In the business sector, diversity in the workforce has become increasingly recognized as a key factor for economic success. According to the *Harvard Business Review*, diversity in leadership is a means to unlocking innovation. Their research suggests that employees of companies with diverse leaders are 45% more likely to report market growth. These employees are also 70% more likely to report that their company captured new markets compared with employees of companies whose leadership lacks diversity [2]. McKinsey & Company, a management consulting firm for 80% of the world's largest corporations, recently published data reaffirming the correlation between diversity in the workplace and financial outperformance. They found that companies in the top quartile for gender and ethnic diversity on their executive teams were more likely to experience above-average profitability than companies in the bottom quartile for these measures of diversity (Fig. 1). Furthermore, they reported that companies in the fourth quartile for both gender and ethnic diversity were more likely to underperform their industry peers by 29% on profitability [4].

Despite this evidence for the benefits of workforce diversity and improved inclusion in leadership positions, companies have struggled to achieve equal representation, especially in leadership. Approximately 39% of the US population belong to minority ethnic and racial groups. In contrast, only 11% to 12% of executive positions are held by ethnically diverse individuals (Fig. 2). To further describe the lack of ethnic and cultural diversity in industry leadership, McKinsey & Company reports that although 10% of US college graduates are black, black Americans hold only 4% of US company executive positions. Hispanic/Latino Americans comprise 8% of graduates and only 4% of executives, and Asian Americans 7% of graduates compared with 5% of executives [4].

DIVERSITY IN MEDICINE

While the nation's demographics shift toward increased diversification, women and people from racial and ethnic minority groups continue to face underrepresentation in the medical workforce similar to their lack of representation in business. The Association of American Medical Colleges (AAMC) defines underrepresentation in medicine as "those racial and ethnic populations that are underrepresented in the medical profession relative to their number in the general population" [5]. Women make up 50.8% and minorities (ie, African American/black, Asian, Hispanic/Latino, American Indian/Alaska Native, or Native Hawaiian/Pacific Islander) make up approximately 39% of the US

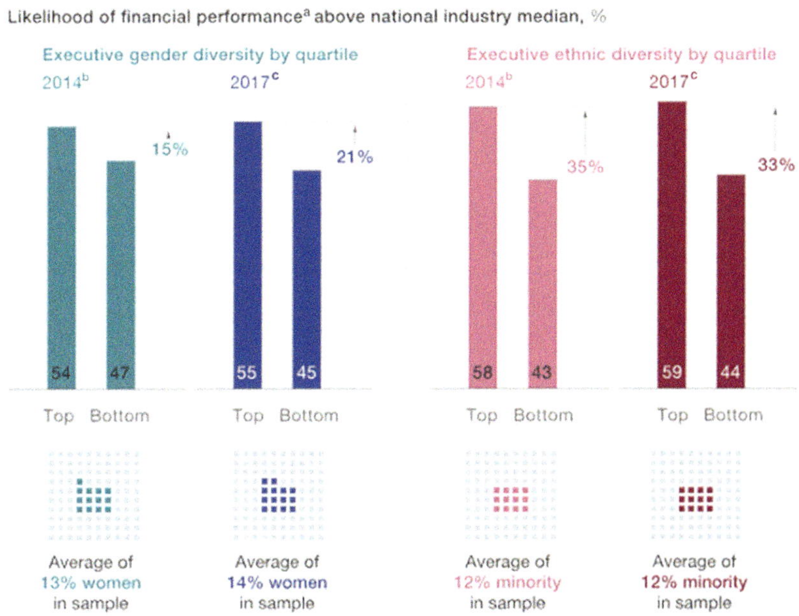

Fig. 1. Companies in the top quartile of gender and ethnic diversity in their leadership teams continue to be significantly more profitable than companies with the lowest quartile of gender diversity. This finding is represented by the bars in likelihood of financial performance greater than the mean. Despite this, the percentages of women and minorities in leadership continue to lag, as the matrix graphs below the bars reveal. [a] Average earnings-before-interest-and-taxes margin, 2010 to 2013 in Diversity Matters 1 and 2011 to 2015 in Diversity Matters II. [b] Results are statistically significant at $P<.10$. [c] Results are statistically significant at $P<.05$. (Exhibits from "Delivering through Diversity", January 2018, McKinsey & Company, www.mckinsey.com. Reprinted by permission.)

population [6]. However, in medicine, minorities represent only 8.9% of the current US physician workforce [7]. Although 2018 marked the first year ever that the number of women applicants and matriculants in US medical schools exceeded the number of male enrollees, women in medicine continue to struggle to achieve career and academic advancement that is similar to their male colleagues [8].

The representation of women in US medical school faculty (39%) is much less than their representation in the population as a whole [9]. However, the disproportionate number of women faculty grows more unequal in academic leadership roles. Only 9.2% of all chairpersons and 9.3% of medical school deans are women. Likewise, minorities are also underrepresented in academic medicine and struggle to attain leadership roles. People from ethnic and racial minority groups represent only 6% of academic chairs and 7.8% of medical school deans [10]. Furthermore, studies have shown that women and minorities are less likely to be promoted to the rank of associate or full professor than male academic physicians who are white [8].

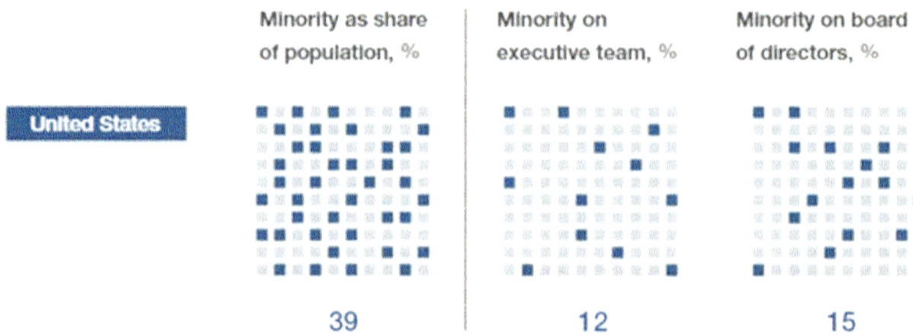

Fig. 2. Executive ethnic diversity relative to population diversity in the United States. Ethnic minority is defined as black/African American, Hispanic/Latino, Asian, Pacific Islander, Native American, mixed race, and other nonwhite ethnicities. (Exhibits from "Delivering through Diversity", January 2018, McKinsey & Company, www.mckinsey.com. Copyright ©2019 McKinsey & Company. All rights reserved. Reprinted by permission.)

Lack of diversity in the medical workforce has been described as a potential contributing factor to the disparities in US health care that have been well documented for many years. Patients representing minority groups have worse measures of health care quality and poorer access to care than their white counterparts [11]. People living in rural areas are less likely to receive preventive care and more likely to experience language barriers than those living in urban communities. White patients living in high socioeconomic status areas have longer life expectancy after an acute myocardial infarction than minority patient and patients living in low socioeconomic status areas [12]. Eight percent of individuals identifying as lesbian, gay, or bisexual, and 27% of transgender or gender-nonconforming individuals report being refused care because of their gender identity/sexual orientation [13]. However, anesthesiology is not immune to disparities in patient care. Studies have shown that black, Hispanic, Medicaid, and/or uninsured patients may be less likely to receive regional anesthesia during hip and knee replacement surgery [14] and that black and Hispanic women are less likely than white women to receive epidural analgesia for labor [15].

DIVERSITY IN ANESTHESIOLOGY

Not dissimilar from the medical field in general, the US anesthesiology workforce has historically been dominated by white men, who represented approximately 54.7% of US anesthesiologists in 2013 [7]. The representation of women in anesthesiology has slowly increased over time, from 22% in 2007 to 24.8% in 2013 [16]. However, this proportion still lags significantly behind the 38% of the general medical workforce who are women and even more so behind the gender diversity of the current US population. Black physicians represent 4.2% of anesthesiologists, on par with the general medical workforce, but in stark contrast to US population demographics, of which blacks/African Americans represent 13%. Combined, minorities (African American/black, Asian, Hispanic/Latino, American Indian/Alaska Native, and Native

Hawaiian/Pacific Islander) make up 39% of the US population and only 20.3% of anesthesiologist in the United States [7].

Themes of underrepresentation of women and racial/ethnic minorities in anesthesiology are also present in the anesthesia subspecialties. Pain medicine ranks among the bottom quartile of medical specialties in terms of female applicants, female trainees, and proportion of female practitioners [17]. At present, women represent approximately 23.2% of trainees in pain medicine [8]. The proportion of female anesthesia critical care fellows has significantly increased from 11.6% to 27.0% over 10 years (2004–2014), a fraction that more closely parallels the representation of women in the general medical workforce [17]. However, minority representation in critical care has seen less growth. Critical care trainees identifying as black represent only 3.9%, Hispanic fellows represent 8.4%, and American Indian/Alaskan Native/Native Hawaiian/Pacific Islander fellows only 0.3%. Compared with US population demographics, these data signify significant underrepresentation of women and minorities in critical care fellowship training programs.

As the aforementioned lack of diversity in anesthesiology has become increasingly identified, calls for improved workforce diversity have amplified across the country. These calls have resulted in an increase, albeit a slow increase, in the number of women and underrepresented minorities in the practice of academic anesthesiology. However, the improvement in representation has not been met with improved inclusion in leadership. Mirroring the general medical workforce, women and minorities in academic anesthesiology departments have not had the same success in obtaining professional advancement as their white male counterparts (Fig. 3). Seventy-five percent of women in

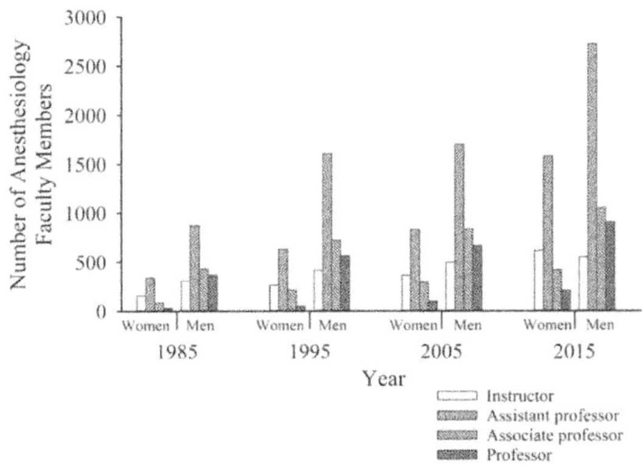

Fig. 3. Distribution of academic ranks among women and men anesthesiology faculty members, 1985 to 2015. The distribution of academic ranks among women anesthesiology faculty members has remained unchanged from 2005 to 2015 (*P* = .27). (*From* Bissing MA, Lange EMS1 Davila WF, et al. Status of Women in Academic Anesthesiology: A 10-Year Update. Anesth Analg. 2019 Jan;128(1):137-143. https://doi.org/10.1213/ANE.0000000000003691.)

academic anesthesiology departments hold junior faculty positions (instructor or assistant professor) and only 6.9% hold full professor appointments [18].

Regarding leadership in academic anesthesiology, most (89.6%) anesthesiology department chairs are men. Furthermore, most anesthesiology department chairs are white, and minority groups only hold 12.3% of these leadership positions. Minorities are more poorly represented as department chairs in anesthesiology than as department chairs across all specialties, where they make up 18.9%. Furthermore, only 3.8% of anesthesiology department chairs are minority women [9]. In addition, women made up only 31% of US anesthesiology residency program directors in 2017, and this underrepresentation has been unchanged since 2009 [19].

The American Society of Anesthesiologists (ASA) is the primary organization that represents physician anesthesiologists in the United States. This organization is one of the leading patient safety organizations in the country and creates clinical guidelines in addition to specialty-wide initiatives that shape the global practice of anesthesiology. Its governing body, the House of Delegates, acts as the leadership group that holds the keys to decision making for the ASA as a whole. A recent study by Toledo and colleagues [3] (2017) surveyed the ASA leadership to evaluate the gender and racial/ethnic diversity within this group. They reported that women and minorities are underrepresented in the leadership of the ASA, with women making up 21.1% and minorities 6.0% of the House of Delegates. Both proportions lag behind the fraction of women and minorities in the general anesthesia workforce (25% and 8.6%, respectively), the national medical workforce (38% and 8.9%), and the US population (50.8% and 32%).

CURRENT EFFORTS TO IMPROVE DIVERSITY AND INCLUSION

In alignment with corporate's evolving understanding of the benefits of workplace diversity, medical organizations are also embracing workforce diversity and inclusion as a means to address health care disparities and improve health care overall. In their 2016 "Resource Paper: Supporting Diversity in the Health Professions," the Council on Graduate Medical Education (COGME) [20] and the Health Resources and Services Administration (HRSA) state that expanding workforce diversity in health care could lead to greater access to care for underserved populations and better interpersonal interactions between patients and health professionals.

Research suggests that minority patients tend to receive better interpersonal care with improved patient satisfaction rates when they interact with medical providers of their own race or ethnicity. Non–English-speaking patients show greater medical comprehension and adherence to follow-up recommendations when patient-provider language concordance exists [21]. Underrepresented minority medical professionals have been shown to be more likely to serve racial and ethnic minority populations in underserved communities [22]. Furthermore, expanding diversity in the medical workforce has the potential to promote participation of underserved populations in clinical studies, improving the ability to provide excellence in health care. Much of the business case for diversification of the medical workforce stems from translating the positive correlation with workforce diversity and patient satisfaction into satisfaction-centered reimbursement models. Overall, increasing diversity and inclusion in medicine has the potential to increase value and reduce costs.

Although diversity and inclusion are terms that have recently gained traction in headlines, efforts to cultivate a more diverse medical workforce are not new. Dating back to 1964, the Student National Medical Association (SNMA) is a national organization with local chapters at both allopathic and osteopathic medical schools across the country. The core mission of this organization is committed to "supporting current and future underrepresented minority medical students, addressing the needs of underserved communities, and increasing the number of clinically excellent, culturally competent and socially conscious physicians" [23]. SNMA has grown in size and support over the years and remains active in fostering diversity and inclusion in medicine. More recently, many programs and initiatives have been developed by academic institutions and professional organizations to continue progress and improve inclusion. Numerous diversity and inclusion committees have been formed in academic departments, training programs, and medical societies. Programs to encourage recruitment of a diverse future generation of physicians have flourished and scholarships/loans for medical students from disadvantaged backgrounds have multiplied [20].

Like the SNMA's many outreach programs, efforts to expose the nation's youth who come from diverse backgrounds to anesthesiology have been developed. The goal: recruiting a more diverse medical school applicant pool with interests in anesthesia and perioperative care. The ASA Committee on Professional Diversity has partnered with the American Medical Association (AMA) to hold the Doctors Back to School Program. Through this pipeline exposure program, anesthesiologists from different minority groups visit youth classrooms annually to talk to children about medicine and anesthesiology. This program aims to get children from underrepresented backgrounds interested in anesthesia and show that this is an attainable career goal through introducing the children to anesthesiologists who look just like them and come from similar backgrounds [24].

The Women in Anesthesiology (WIA) organization was recently established by Dr Rekha Chandrabose, who obtained a small grant through the ASA's Committee on Professional Diversity. WIA was created to promote the professional development of women physician anesthesiologists [25]. This organization was instrumental in advocating for the American Board of Anesthesiology (ABA) 2019 policy change regarding resident absence from training that exceeds 60 working days [26]. One benefit of this policy may be improved inclusion of resident physicians with diverse training paths caused by parental leave, family leave, or medical illness.

The Society for Neuroscience in Anesthesiology and Critical Care (SNACC) published a diversity initiative for their organization in 2017. Within this initiative, potential action items included establishing a diversity committee and a diversity mentorship program. In addition, a mission statement was created that states, "SNACC members are committed to individual and organizational efforts to welcome a diverse group of scientists and practitioners and safeguard fairness, equality, and respect" [27]. SNACC has made additional efforts to encourage organizational diversity and inclusion, including the creation of the Women in Neuroanesthesiology and Neuroscience Education and Research (WINNER) program. This program celebrates successful women in neuroanesthesia and aims to provide support, mentorship, and sponsorship for early-career and midcareer women in anesthesiology [28].

FUTURE STRATEGIES TO IMPROVE DIVERSITY AND INCLUSION

The business strategies to push innovation and growth through increasing diversity and inclusion can serve as a model for medicine. The first steps include leadership commitment to diversity and inclusion. CEO Action for Diversity and Inclusion is a business community endeavor to collectively advance diversity and inclusion, including sharing of strategies and collective accountability [29]. One business example of successful diversification and inclusion is IBM, whose CEO targeted identifying issues in various groups and addressing them to increase women and minorities in leadership positions, which has led to the ability to find new markets and drive growth [30].

Promotion of diversity in medicine and specifically anesthesiology will create a physician cohort that is able to collaboratively innovate and adapt to the future. As has been proved in business, actively seeking diversity will allow adaption to changes in the field and in the patients that are served.

Several specialties have created pathways to increase diversity [31,32]. One option is to create avenues for early exposure to anesthesia in medical school, with voluntary selective time with anesthesiologists, and information sessions about the specialty. Summer internship programs have been used in other specialties to provide further opportunities [33]. Mentors for women and minorities who show interest will allow ongoing exposure and can lead to more competitive applicants.

Academic anesthesia departments can create policies to actively consider women and minorities for open positions. Improving opportunities for women and minorities to advance can be provided by active mentorship and sponsorship for junior faculty. A family-friendly departmental environment that encourages things such as committee meetings at optimal times and childcare at national meetings can limit loss of peer support and encourage engagement after a leave is taken.

SUMMARY

Although much work is yet to be done, progress toward training a more diverse and inclusive future medical workforce has occurred. As previously noted, most medical students are now women, with 53.4% of matriculating students in 2018 being women according to the AAMC Annual Student

Questionnaire [32]. These data also showed growth in the representation of minority medical students that now seems to be mirroring changes in US population demographics. Forty-five percent of medical students matriculating in 2018 self-identified their race/ethnicity as belonging to a minority group (American Indian/Alaska Native 0.9%, Asian 24.5%, black/African American 8.3%, Hispanic/Latino 11.0%, Native Hawaiian/Pacific Islander 0.3%). Approximately 7.7% of matriculated medical students reported being bisexual, gay, or lesbian, and 0.7% reported identifying with a gender that is different from their sex assigned at birth.

Trends of increasing gender diversity in the future medical workforce have also been observed in anesthesiology training programs, in which 36.8% of residents are women [9]. Against the changing backdrop of national population demographics in the United States, the lack of diversity and inclusion among anesthesiologists has the potential to magnify health care disparities, adversely affect outcomes, depress patient satisfaction scores, and negatively affect reimbursement.

Fostering further progress to expand the diversity of physicians trained in anesthesiology has the potential to bolster scientific innovation, increase participation of underrepresented populations in clinical studies and thus increase the likelihood that research outcomes will benefit underserved individuals, and expand public trust in the health care system [34]. Ultimately, moving toward greater diversity in anesthesiology may allow the optimization of perioperative outcomes, similar to the gains that COGME aims to achieve in improving care for all.

References

[1] Hewlett SA, Marshall M, Sherbin L. How diversity can drive innovation. Harvard Business Review 2013.

[2] News Census Bureau Report Analyzes U.S. Population projections. Washington, DC: U.S. Census Bureau Public Information Office; 2015. Available at: https://www.census.gov/newsroom/press-release/2015/cb15-tps16.html. Accessed March 12, 2019.

[3] Toledo P, Duce L, Adams J, et al. Diversity in the American Society of Anesthesiologists leadership. Anesth Analg 2017;124(5):1611–6.

[4] Delivering through diversity. McKinsey and Company; 2018. Available at: https://www.mckinsey.com/business-functions/organization/our-insights/delivering-through-diversity. Accessed February 19, 2019.

[5] Association of American Medical Colleges. Underrepresented in medicine definition 2003. Available at: https://www.aamc.org/initiatives/urm/. Accessed April 10, 2019.

[6] Quick Facts from the US Census Bureau. 2018. Available at: http://www.census.gov/quickfacts/fact/table/US/PST045218. Accessed April 5, 2019.

[7] Diversity in the physician workforce: facts and figures. Available at: https://www.aamc.org/data/workforce/reports/439214/workforcediversity.html. Accessed April 5, 2019.

[8] Association of American Medical Colleges. More women than men enrolled in US medical schools in 2017 2017. Available at: https://news.aamc.org/press-release/article/applicant-enrollment-2017/. Accessed April 5, 2019.

[9] The state of women in academic medicine: the pipeline and pathways to leadership 2015-2016. Available at: https://www.aamc.org/members/gwims/statistics/489870/stats16.html. Accessed April 5, 2019.

[10] Yu PT, Parsa PV, Hassanein O, et al. Minorities struggle to advance in academic medicine: a 12 year review of diversity at the highest levels of American's teaching institutions. J Surg Res 2013;182:212–8.
[11] 2017 National Healthcare Disparities Report. Agency for healthcare research and quality Rockville (MD). Available at: https://www.ahrq.gov/research/findings/nhqrdr/nhqdr17/index.html. Accessed April 8, 2019.
[12] American Heart Association Statistics Committee and Stroke Statistics Subcommittee. Heart disease and stroke statistics-2019 update: a report from the American Heart Association Statistics Committee and Stroke Statistics Subcommittee. Circulation 2019;139(10): e56–528.
[13] Lambda Legal. When health care isn't caring: Lambda Legal's survey of discrimination against LGBT people and people living with HIV. New York: Lambda Legal; 2010.
[14] Minority, medicaid hip and knee replacement patients less likely to received regional anesthesia. 2015. Available at: https://www.asahq.org/about-asa/newsroom/news-releases/2015/10/minorities-less-likely-get-regional-anest. Accessed March 25, 2019.
[15] Glance LG, Wissler R, Glantz C, et al. Racial differences in the use of epidural analgesia for labor. Anesthesiology 2007;106(1):19–25.
[16] Baird M, Daugherty L, Kumar KB, et al. Regional and gender differences and trends in the anesthesiologist workforce. Anesthesiology 2015;123:997–1012.
[17] Doshi TL, Bicket MC. Why aren't there more female pain medicine physicians? Reg Anesth Pain Med 2018;43(5):516–20.
[18] Bissing MA, Lange EMS, Davila WF, et al. Status of women in academic anesthesiology: a 10-year update. Anesth Analg 2019;128(1):137–43.
[19] Kenevan MR, Stewart TM, Warner MA, et al. The changing characteristics of anesthesiology program directors. J Educ Perioper Med 2018;20(3):E625.
[20] Council on Graduate Medical Education. Resource paper: supporting diversity in the health professions. 2016. Available at: https://www.hrsa.gov/advisorycommittees/bhpradvisory/cogme/Publications/diversityresourcepaper.pdf. Accessed March 23, 2019.
[21] DuVivier D. Addressing health care inequities through increased diversity and inclusion in academic anesthesiology programs. ASA Newsl 2017;81(5):54–6.
[22] Department of Health and Human Services, Health Resources and Services Administration, Bureau of Health Professions. The rationale for diversity in the health professions: a review of the evidence. Rockville (MD): HHS (US); 2006.
[23] The Student National Medical Association. 2019. Available at: http://www.snma.org/. Accesse April 14, 2019.
[24] Kreso M, Young Anderson B, Bradley SL, et al. Because we could, ASA pipeline to anesthesia. ASA Monitor 2018;82(2):56–7.
[25] Women in anesthesiology. 2019. Available at: https://www.womeninanesthesiology.org. Accessed April 15, 2019.
[26] The American Board of Anesthesiology. Absence from training policy guidelines. 2019. Available at: http://www.theaba.org/PDFs/BOI/Absence-from-Training-Policy-Guidelines. Accessed April 15, 2019.
[27] Diversity Initiative for SNACC. Society for neuroscience in anesthesiology and critical care 2017. Available at: https://www.snacc.org/wp-content/upoads/2017/fall/article3.html. Accessed April 5, 2019.
[28] Sharma D. Celebrating exceptional women leaders and mentoring the next generation: The WINNER (Women in Neuroanesthesiology & Neuroscience Education & Research) Program. ASA Newsl 2018;82(8):56–7.
[29] CEO ActIon for diversity and inclusion. Available at: https://www.ceoaction.com/. Accessed April 15, 2019.
[30] Thomas DA. Diversity as Strategy. Available at: https://hbr.org/2004/09/diversity-as-strategy. Accessed April 8, 2019.

[31] Lightfoote JB, Deville D, Ma LD, et al. Diversity, inclusion, and representation: it is time to act. J Am Coll Radiol 2016;13:1421–5.
[32] Association of American Medical Colleges. Matriculating student questionnaire 2018. Available at: https://www.aamc.org/data/msq/. Accessed April 10, 2019.
[33] Mason BS, Ross W, Ortega G, et al. Can a strategic pipeline initiative increase the number of women and underrepresented minorities in orthopaedic surgery? Clin Orthop Relat Res 2016;474:1979–85.
[34] Diversity in extramural programs. National Institutes of Health; 2019. Available at: http://www.extramural-diversity.nih.gov. Accessed April 15, 2019.

INTRODUCTION

The origin story of the opioid epidemic cataclysm is one of greed, misunderstanding, and unintended consequences [1]. This story of opioid abuse is also one that is well-known not just within the medical community, but also to our patients. Driving this awareness of the opioid abuse pandemic is an interplay between the current political climate, editor proxy, global events, advertiser's influence, social media, and personal events. We are perpetually inundated on the evening news or on social media regarding rising opioid deaths and there is increasing focus on legislation at the state and federal levels to put an end to the opioid crisis.

In 2017, more than 47,000 people in the United States died after an opioid overdose. This works out to 1 person dying every 11 minutes from a preventable and catastrophic death. In that same year, 1.7 million United States citizens suffered from a substance abuse disorder related to prescription opioids and 652,000 abused heroin [2,3]. According to data from the Centers for Disease Control and Prevention, drug overdose death rates in the United States have experienced a 4-fold increase between 1999 and 2017 with the greatest increase occurring in males and those between the ages of 25 and 65 years [4]. The impact of the large number of premature deaths related to opioid administration is one of the primary factors related to the decrease in overall life expectancy reported in 2017 [5]. Although there are no opioids that are entirely without blame, synthetic opioids and heroin are largely responsible for the increase in observed age-adjusted drug overdose death rates secondary to opioids [4].

If one examines only the economic burden of opioid-related abuse, the estimates of annual costs from calendar year 2013 in the United States are $78.5 billion. These costs were related to the provision of health care, lost productivity, addiction treatment, and the criminal justice system [6]. Given the growth of this problem, it is likely that annual costs will continue to increase and, without intervention, might very well overwhelm our health care system.

Behind all the staggering numerical data, there are patients longing for treatment of both their chronic disease and for acute pain management after surgical procedures in the setting of either opioid tolerance or opioid antagonists. These patients may be challenging to treat and may suffer from several comorbid psychiatric and medical conditions. Compounding the problem for patients with a history of chronic pain is that they may experience marginalization at the hands of health care providers and may subsequently harbor sentiments that make them less likely to trust health care providers in the future [7,8].

Patients with chronic pain or those who go on to develop persistent postsurgical pain may also be at increased risk for the development of postoperative complications or increased costs related to treatment of a variety of potential complications or prolonged hospital admissions [9,10]. However, a thorough and compassionate strategy that avoids marginalization of patient concerns is the best approach to improve patient satisfaction while simultaneously maximizing outcomes. We have progressed a long way since the outdated mantra of stamping out pain and overemphasizing pain as the fifth vital sign. However, we need to recognize that the medical community contributed to the rate of opioid use and abuse disorders and that we need to have a systematic approach to management that emphasizes quality, cost-effective, and compassionate care. Patients undergoing treatment for opioid use or abuse disorders may be difficult to manage in the perioperative setting and therefore consideration should be given to evidence-based, multidisciplinary care to maximize success. The focus of this article is an overview of the medications currently approved for medication-assisted therapy (MAT) to help patients manage substance abuse disorder and the perioperative analgesic approach for these patients.

BUPRENORPHINE

Available since the 1970s, buprenorphine has been used as both an alternative to methadone in the treatment of opioid dependence and as an adjunct in chronic pain management. Buprenorphine is a partial agonist of the mu opioid receptor and an antagonist of the kappa opioid receptor. With activation of the mu opioid receptor, buprenorphine provides analgesia similar to full mu opioid receptor agonists. However, secondary to partial agonist activity at these receptors, the dose–response curve plateaus such that respiratory depression is unlikely [11]. This ceiling effect at higher doses makes buprenorphine an ideal agent for chronic pain management in opioid-dependent or -tolerant patients [12,13]. Buprenorphine has the highest affinity for the mu receptor of all opioids and will therefore displace and prevent binding of the mu receptor by concurrently administered full opioid agonists. It is metabolized hepatically via the cytochrome P-450 CYP3A4 system and has an active metabolite, norbuprenorphine, which has one-fifth the activity of buprenorphine [14]. In addition, the dissociation rate of buprenorphine from the mu receptor is approximately 166 minutes and the half-life is between 25 and 48 hours; thus, it takes 2 to 3 days for this agent to be eliminated from the body [15]. This long elimination half-life has implications for those patients treated with buprenorphine formulations who present for surgery expected to result in significant perioperative pain.

Buprenorphine is available in multiple formulations including sublingual, buccal, transdermal, and implantable or injectable formulations either alone or in combination with naloxone (Table 1). The addition of naloxone to buprenorphine formulations further decreases the abuse potential of this agent because naloxone blocks the euphoric effects of opioids if injected parenterally.

With increasing rates of opioid use disorders in the United States, the number of patients treated with buprenorphine and the number of prescribers providing buprenorphine are experiencing tremendous growth. Under the Drug Addiction Treatment Act of 2000, prescribers are required to undergo an 8-hour class to be eligible to prescribe buprenorphine and can apply for waivers to increase the number of patients that can be treated by each provider. There are more than 14,000 prescribers under Medicare Part D. Claims made by these prescribers for buprenorphine containing medications have increased

Table 1
Available formulations of buprenorphine, methadone, and naltrexone

Brand name	Generic name	Formulation
Belbuca	Buprenorphine	Transbuccal
Buprenex	Buprenorphine	IV or IM injection
Butrans	Buprenorphine	Transdermal patch
Probuphine	Buprenorphine	Implant
Subutex	Buprenorphine	Sublingual
Suboxone	Buprenorphine with naloxone	Sublingual
Zubsolv	Buprenorphine with naloxone	Sublingual
Dolophine, Methadose	Methadone	PO
Methadone HCl Intensol	Methadone	PO solution
(No brand name)	Methadone	IV
ReVia	Naltrexone	PO
Vivitrol	Naltrexone	Intramuscular

Abbreviations: IM, intramuscular; IV, intravenous; PO, orally.
Data from Lexicomp Online (Lexi-Drugs, UW Health Formulary), Hudson, Ohio: Wolters Kluwer Clinical Drug Information, Inc.; 2013; April 15, 2013.

from 26,400 in 2011 to 90,900 in 2015 [16]. Hence, there is an increasing likelihood that anesthesia providers will encounter patients chronically consuming buprenorphine for either chronic pain or abuse disorders. Therefore, it is imperative that anesthesia providers understand the mechanism of action for buprenorphine and have developed a plan for the perioperative management of these patients.

PERIOPERATIVE MANAGEMENT

There is no consensus on the perioperative management of patients treated with buprenorphine and most published recommendations are derived from expert opinion or individual case reports. Perioperative management strategies should not be developed or implemented in a vacuum or anesthesia-dominated silo. Continuous involvement of patients and their buprenorphine prescribers is essential to minimize the risk of opioid relapse or overdose and improve the likelihood of providing perioperative analgesia.

One strategy is simply the continuation of perioperative buprenorphine and encouraging patients to administer their usual morning dose before any planned surgical procedure. Support for this approach was provided by several recently published meta-analyses. These studies have demonstrated a detrimental analgesic effect related to discontinuing buprenorphine therapy in the perioperative period, especially when patients are maintained on lower doses (ie, <16 mg/d) [17,18]. It is important to recall that buprenorphine possesses significant agonist activity. Therefore, if patients discontinue their buprenorphine therapy preoperatively, they have been found to suffer through increased pain and require significantly more opioids in the first 24 hours after surgery than those who are continued on their buprenorphine preoperatively [19].

Should buprenorphine therapy be continued, different dosing strategies may result in reasonable postoperative outcomes. In select patients, maintenance of home dosing regimens, supplemented with multimodal and opioid analgesics, may be appropriate. In other patients, the analgesic impact of buprenorphine therapy can be exploited to provide postoperative analgesia and increases in buprenorphine may be beneficial [18]. Any changes in buprenorphine therapy need to be done in concert with the patient's primary buprenorphine provider.

An alternative strategy would be to decrease the preoperative dose of buprenorphine with the hope that a decreased buprenorphine dose may increase opioid receptor availability for full opioid agonists [20]. Other, less used, strategies include converting the patient's buprenorphine needs to a short-acting full agonist opioid or methadone therapy. These changes would need to be done with the full participation of the patient's primary buprenorphine prescriber and variabilities in opioid conversions and cross-tolerance would need to be considered. Patients receiving injectable or implantable buprenorphine therapy will need to be treated similarly to those patients whose oral buprenorphine therapy has been continued throughout the perioperative process.

Protocols have been developed that have attempted to make a distinction between the acuity of surgery, the expected postoperative analgesic requirements, and the daily dose of buprenorphine. The first well-established protocol for these patients was developed at the University of Michigan and was intended to address the analgesic needs for those patients consuming buprenorphine in the setting of chronic pain management. In this protocol, patients undergoing surgical procedures expected to result in minimal postoperative pain are treated with continuation of buprenorphine therapy. For elective surgical procedures expected to result in moderate to severe postoperative pain, the protocol suggests transitioning buprenorphine therapy to a short-acting full opioid agonist. When patients consuming buprenorphine present for emergent surgery, the buprenorphine should be discontinued after surgery, and a multimodal regimen should be implemented [21].

With this protocol in mind, if the perioperative analgesic plan calls for buprenorphine therapy to be paused, the significant elimination time of this medication requires stopping the medication 48 to 72 hours before surgery [22]. This protocol also recommends that the duration of buprenorphine cessation before surgery be based on the patient's dose of buprenorphine; those on a low dose of 0 to 4 mg/d should pause therapy for 24 hours, whereas those on a moderate or high dose of greater than 8 mg/d should hold for 72 hours. In patients with implantable formulations, removing the implanted drug may not be realistic, and these patients will likely present difficulties with opioid-based postoperative analgesic regimens [21].

The decision to continue or stop buprenorphine therapy in the perioperative period is not one to be taken lightly. Reasons for this are numerous, but chief among them is that there is an increase in mortality in the first 4 weeks after cessation of buprenorphine treatment [23]. In patients with a history of depression, anxiety, or substance abuse, the decision to discontinue buprenorphine is not without risk. In all patients on buprenorphine, not specifically limited to those in the perioperative period, discontinuing buprenorphine led to at least a 50% relapse in opioid use [24]. Decisions regarding changes to a patient's buprenorphine dosing must be done in conjunction with the patient, surgeon, anesthesiologist, and primary prescriber. See Fig. 1 for a potential algorithm to help initiate the development of a preliminary perioperative plan.

Overall, maximizing perioperative multimodal analgesia and regional anesthesia techniques may offer perioperative benefits. In addition, using a collaborative acute pain management consult service that involves representatives from anesthesiology, pharmacy, physical therapy, addiction medicine, and psychiatry may offer contributions to perioperative pain management.

Finally, after surgery and discharge from the hospital, a concrete plan needs to be in place to ensure a smooth transition back to buprenorphine therapy. Restarting buprenorphine in the setting of high doses of full opioid agonists could precipitate acute withdrawal. Buprenorphine should be restarted 12 to 24 hours after a dose of a short-acting opioid such as oxycodone and 24 to 48 hours after a dose of a long-acting opioid such as morphine [11]. Consideration should be given to restarting buprenorphine at a low dose of 1 to 2 mg/d and up titrating back to the preoperative dose over 1 to 2 days while closely observing for signs of withdrawal [11].

METHADONE

Methadone is approved by the US Food and Drug Administration for maintenance therapy in the setting of opioid use disorder and in the treatment of moderate to severe chronic pain. Methadone is also gaining popularity for acute

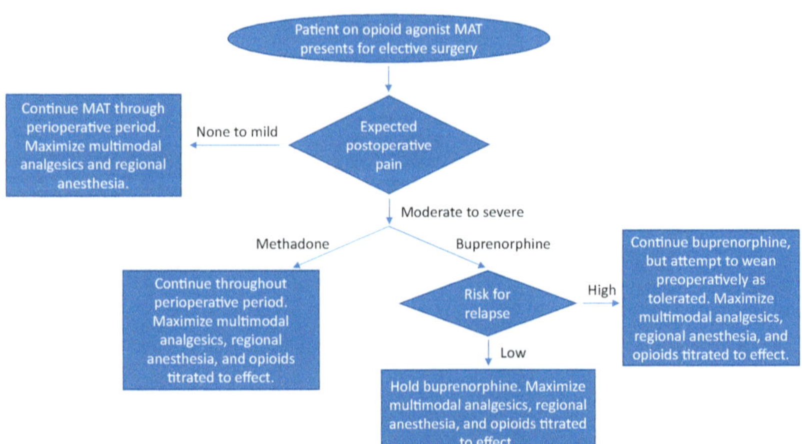

Fig. 1. Potential algorithm to help initiate the development of a perioperative pain management plan for patients on opioid agonist MAT (buprenorphine or methadone).

pain management in the perioperative setting for patients expected to experience significant postoperative pain [25,26]. Ambulatory dosing strategies are based on the indication as the analgesic effects of methadone are related to the alpha-elimination phase whereas the withdrawal suppression is related to the beta-elimination phase [27]. As such, methadone is usually administered multiple times per day if being prescribed for chronic pain and only once daily when prescribed for MAT [27,28]. Providers who prescribe methadone must have a separate Drug Enforcement Administration registration as an opioid treatment program, which also needs to be certified by Substance Abuse and Mental Health Services Administration.

Methadone is a diphenylpropylamine opioid that is a racemic mixture of 2 enantiomers. The R-methadone enantiomer is a full mu opioid receptor agonist. The S-methadone enantiomer has N-methyl-D-aspartate (NMDA) antagonist and serotonin and norepinephrine reuptake blocking properties [27,28]. Methadone is metabolized by the hepatic cytochrome P450 system. The main metabolite formed is inactive, but there are 2 minor metabolites (methadol and normethadol) that behave similarly to methadone [28]. The half-life of methadone ranges from 8 to 59 hours, but in patients with impaired hepatic function, methadone may accumulate, and exaggerated or prolonged effects may be encountered. Methadone is ultimately excreted via the fecal and renal routes, where renal excretion of unchanged drug typically accounts for less than 10% of elimination. Notably, methadone is not dialyzable [29].

Methadone is available in tablet, soluble tablet, solution, and injectable formulations (see Table 1). As a tablet or oral solution, it has up to 95% bioavailability. The duration of action is anywhere from 4 to 8 hours after a single dose to 22 to 48 hours after multiple doses [29].

There are multiple important factors to consider when initiating methadone owing to its unique pharmacologic profile. Before initiation, it is recommended to wean down or off other opioids, if possible, because initiating methadone therapy in the setting of other opioids increases the risk of adverse side effects. Methadone has a long and variable half-life, so multiple days are required to reach a steady-state concentration. Thus, care should be taken with initiation and up-titration of methadone. There is interpatient variability in absorption, duration of action, and elimination. This may be partly because methadone can accumulate in multiple tissues after multiple doses and subsequently be slowly released, thus, variably prolonging the duration of action [29,30].

Methadone has a higher binding affinity for the mu opioid receptor than morphine [31]. Therefore, when patients maintained on chronic methadone abuse heroin, which is metabolized to morphine, the euphoric effects are attenuated. There continues to be an increased risk for respiratory depression when methadone is combined with heroin as methadone does not occupy 100% of the mu opioid receptors at the typical doses given for treatment of substance abuse disorder [28]. Similar interactions occur when methadone is administered alongside short-acting opioids in the setting of acute postoperative pain.

PERIOPERATIVE MANAGEMENT

Because methadone is a full mu opioid agonist, it possesses significant analgesic properties. These patients should be instructed to take their normally prescribed methadone dose the day of their surgical procedure. A reasonable perioperative pain management plan includes continuing methadone and supplementing with immediate-release opioids as needed. Formulating an opioid agreement preoperatively may be helpful because it establishes expectations for the postoperative analgesic course including a plan for discontinuing any short-acting opioids. However, additional opioids should not be the first-line option for these patients. A multimodal approach with nonopioid and nonpharmacologic adjuncts as well as regional anesthesia should be implemented for these patients. In formulating the anesthesia and perioperative pain plan, a recent urine drug screen may be helpful to ensure that methadone has been taken as directed and that other drugs of abuse are not present [28].

Methadone can prolong a patient's QTc, so a recent electrocardiogram should be available before surgery. The QTc should be closely monitored in the perioperative period, especially if additional QTc prolonging medications (eg, droperidol) are administered. It may also be prudent to monitor serum electrolytes, because patients with prolonged QTc are at an increased risk of arrhythmias such as Torsades de pointes, and this risk may be exacerbated by electrolyte abnormalities, especially abnormalities in serum potassium and magnesium levels [28].

Methadone metabolism can be significantly altered by the co-administration of other medications that can impact the CYP450 system. Medications that enhance the hepatic CYP450 system, such as carbamazepine and phenytoin, may decrease plasma levels of methadone. Alternatively, medications that inhibit the CYP450 system, such as fluconazole and ciprofloxacin, could increase the amount of methadone available and cause over-narcotization, especially if given in combination with other opioids in the postoperative setting. Certain commonly prescribed antibiotics, antidepressant, antiepileptic, and antiretroviral medications fall into these categories, so the initiation and discontinuation of these medications should be considered carefully. Although these interactions are possible, they may not necessarily lead to clinically significant effects in every patient. After any medication changes, patients should be monitored, and appropriate adjustments should be made to their methadone dosage [32].

If methadone is discontinued abruptly and not replaced with another opioid during the perioperative period, patients may experience opioid withdrawal. Depending on the indication for methadone, these patients may also be at risk for relapse, so abrupt discontinuation is not recommended.

The perioperative analgesic management of these patients should then be similar to what might be planned for any patient with chronic opioid requirements. Preoperative consultation should focus on the establishment of realistic analgesic goals and treatment options. Analgesic therapy should consist of aggressive efforts to provide multimodal analgesia and continuous regional anesthesia techniques. Methadone therapy should be continued and any changes to the analgesic regimen should be coordinated with the patient's primary opioid prescriber. See Fig. 1 for a potential algorithm to help initiate the development of a preliminary perioperative plan.

NALTREXONE

Naltrexone is approved by the US Food and Drug Administration for MAT of opioid use disorder. This agent differs from methadone and buprenorphine in that it is an opioid antagonist. Therefore, it is recommended that patients are abstinent from opioids for at least 7 to 10 days before initiation of naltrexone therapy to avoid the elicitation of withdrawal symptoms [33]. This pause in opioid administration can be difficult to achieve in this patient population and has been shown to be a barrier to naltrexone initiation, especially in the outpatient setting [34]. However, after overcoming this hurdle, extended-release naltrexone has been shown to be noninferior to buprenorphine in total number of opioid-negative urine tests, days of heroin and other illicit opioid use [35], and relative hazard of relapse [36]. Patients taking extended-release naltrexone also reported a higher percentage of opioid-free weeks and decreased opioid craving when compared with placebo [37]. Treatment with naltrexone may be necessary for patients who have a professional responsibility to avoid opioid agonists (physicians, air traffic controllers, etc). This agent may be slightly easier to obtain because any health care provider who is legally able to prescribe medications can write prescriptions for naltrexone.

Naltrexone is also approved by the US Food and Drug Administration to treat alcohol use disorder. Possibly because of this, alcohol use disorder was 3 times as prevalent among patients who were prescribed naltrexone than those who were prescribed buprenorphine for MAT [38]. Naltrexone is additionally being used in an off-label fashion to lessen the symptoms of fibromyalgia and chronic pain [39,40]. These topics are beyond the scope of this article, but they certainly highlight the diverse patient populations that may present for surgical interventions on naltrexone therapy.

Naltrexone is a cyclopropyl derivative of oxymorphone that acts as a competitive opioid antagonist, especially at the mu opioid receptor. Naltrexone is hepatically metabolized by noncytochrome-mediated dehydrogenase into 6-beta-naexol, an active metabolite, and minor metabolites. A small portion of naltrexone and its metabolites can also undergo glucuronidation. These metabolites and a small portion of unmetabolized naltrexone are primarily excreted in the urine. Oral naltrexone has a half-life of 4 hours and its active metabolite has a half-life of 13 to 14 hours, much longer than naloxone's half-life. Injectable extended-release naltrexone has a half-life of 5 to 10 days [41].

Naltrexone is currently available as an oral tablet and an intramuscular injection (see Table 1). Each tablet is 50 mg and is taken once a day in doses ranging from 50 mg to 150 mg. There is a linear relationship between oral naltrexone dosage and duration of action where each 50 mg lasts for 24 hours [41].

Intramuscular extended-release naltrexone injections contain 380 mg and are released slowly over 4 weeks. Patients receive this injection once a month without any variability in dosing. Although there are 3 brands available, Vivitrol is the only intramuscular formulation approved in the United States [41].

Although oral naltrexone was approved for MAT decades before extended-release naltrexone, a meta-analysis showed oral naltrexone was no more effective than placebo at treating opioid use disorder [42]. Despite this, oral naltrexone was prescribed more frequently than extended-release naltrexone in subsequent years [38]. Thus, patients may continue to be on either oral or injectable naltrexone.

Implantable forms of naltrexone are available but are not commonly prescribed.

As an antagonist, naltrexone blocks the euphoric, analgesic, and sedative effects of opioids, but it can also precipitate withdrawal in patients who have not fully detoxified from opioids. It is not addictive and no physiologic dependence forms. However, after discontinuation of naltrexone, patients may be more sensitive to opioids. Overdose is possible at previously tolerated doses of opioids and therefore close observation is required to ensure that patients do not experience significant respiratory depression [27,43].

PERIOPERATIVE MANAGEMENT

For surgical procedures expected to result in moderate or severe postoperative pain, naltrexone administration should be discontinued in an effort to improve analgesic management. Oral formulations should be held for at least 2 to 3 days and the last dose of the injectable extended release formulation should be 30 days preoperatively [27]. For patients at significant risk for relapse, it is important to coordinate preoperative planning with the patient's naltrexone prescriber. In addition, the patient should be involved in developing the perioperative analgesia plan and should be aware of their increased risk for relapse and difficulties with analgesic management. After discontinuation of naltrexone, patients may experience increased sensitivity to opioids and therefore close monitoring is required to detect respiratory depression [27,43]. Consideration should be given to initiating therapy with lower doses of opioids and titrating to effect once the analgesic, sedative, and respiratory depressant effects have been evaluated. These patients should also have a multimodal analgesic plan, including nonopioid analgesics, nonpharmacologic adjuncts, and continuous regional anesthesia techniques, if appropriate. In the postoperative period, naltrexone should continue to be held until the patient has been opioid free for at least 7 to 10 days to decrease the risk of withdrawal symptoms with the re-initiation of naltrexone [33].

To avoid the risks associated with these periods of time when patients are not taking naltrexone, it may be reasonable to continue this agent for procedures in which little to no pain is expected or where the risk of relapse and overdose is substantially increased. In this situation, it is extremely important that the anesthesia providers and surgical team are aware that the patient will react differently to opioid medications, and they should rely heavily on a multimodal approach to analgesia. It is therefore vital that the surgical team, anesthesia team, and prescribing provider work together to formulate a plan for these patients well before the day of surgery. See Fig. 2 for a potential algorithm to help develop a preliminary perioperative plan for these patients.

If a patient taking naltrexone presents for emergent surgery, it may not be practical to wait until naltrexone has been sufficiently metabolized to allow for opioids to provide effective analgesia. In these scenarios, providers should rely on nonopioid analgesics, nonpharmacologic adjuncts, and continuous regional anesthesia techniques as the foundation of their postoperative pain plan. This is especially true for patients receiving intramuscular naltrexone therapy, because the duration of effect from this route of administration is approximately 4 weeks. If the patient had been taking oral naltrexone, opioid medications could be considered 48 to 72 hours after their last naltrexone dose if pain control remains inadequate. Additionally, naltrexone therapy should continue to be held in the postoperative period until the patient has been opioid free for at least 7 days [33]. Again, multidisciplinary pain management teams can be profoundly helpful in the perioperative management of these patients, especially during the required detoxification period before re-initiation of naltrexone.

THE PERIOPERATIVE SURGICAL HOME

The perioperative surgical home (PSH) emphasizes the benefits that might be realized with a collaborative, interdisciplinary, comprehensive, protocolized, and innovative model of care. PSHs are involved in managing patient care

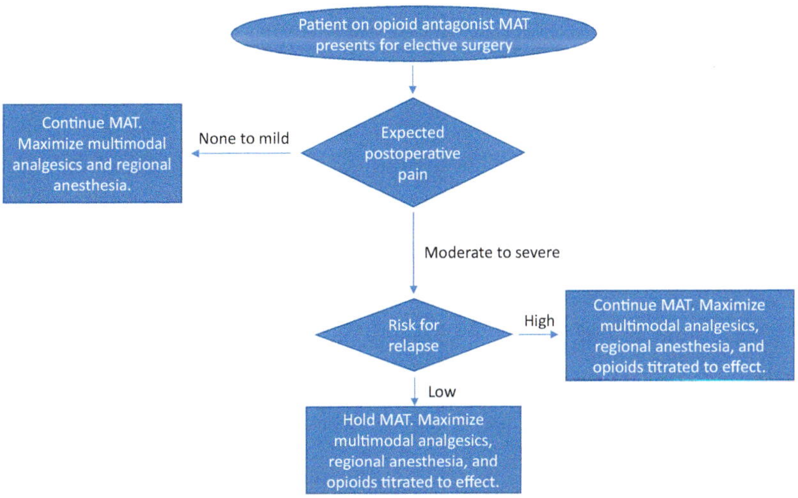

Fig. 2. Potential algorithm to help initiate the development of a perioperative pain management plan for patients on opioid antagonist MAT (naltrexone).

from the time that the decision is made to operate and help to establish the optimal timing of any surgical procedure. The PSH would then coordinate management of all necessary preoperative testing and consults, would ensure that patients are appropriately routed through perioperative pathways (eg, enhanced recovery) and that patients receive evidence-based perioperative management.

With regard to perioperative analgesia, an anesthesia-led PSH and comprehensive perioperative pain service would then be involved in determining a perioperative analgesic plan that would include multimodal preoperative analgesics, regional and neuraxial analgesic techniques, analgesic infusions, and other opioid sparing techniques [44]. This preoperative management may include a preoperative reduction in baseline opioid administration, cessation of opioid antagonists or transitioning from a partial opioid receptor agonist to a full agonist [45]. This model would decrease variability in care, create seamless transitions in patient care, integrate various medical providers, and foster enhanced patient–clinician shared decision making [46]. Broad pain-related management concepts that can be addressed by a well-functioning PSH include emphasizing continuity, coordination, integration, patient-centered and shared decision making, and variability reduction while focusing on improving quality and reducing costs [44].

In the setting of opioid tolerance or history of abuse, the PSH presents an opportunity to deliver patient-centered pain management throughout the perioperative period. These patients need to be identified and met by members of the pain management team before surgery. These visits will help to establish care with the pain management team and allow for the formulation of a perioperative pain management plan. During this initial visit, the patient's history of painful symptoms and medication management (prescriber, medication, dose, frequency, duration, and route) can be discussed. This visit determines if opioid maintenance therapy is prescribed for MAT or analgesic purposes because this information impacts the decision to continue or pause buprenorphine or other opioid antagonist therapies. During this visit, these patients will also have an opportunity to create and take ownership of a personalized perioperative pain management plan. Available multimodal and complementary therapies should be discussed with patients during the preoperative visit. There should also be a discussion about expected postoperative pain levels, how pain exacerbations will be managed, and what the patient's anticipated pain management regimen will be at the time of discharge. Psychological factors that might impact pain management should be addressed, and patients should be allowed an opportunity to discuss relevant fears and anxiety [47].

After the surgery, daily visits by a multidisciplinary pain service will help to provide pain assessments, reinforce and encourage adherence to the predetermined pain regimen, and provide necessary adjustments (Box 1). Members of this multidisciplinary team should include anesthesia pain specialists, but could also include members of the pharmacy, spiritual services, addiction medicine, health psychology, psychiatry, physical medicine and rehabilitation, and

Box 1: A multidisciplinary approach to pain management and patient care is required

Multidisciplinary components required for patients on MAT

- Medication-assisted treatment prescriber
- Anesthesia providers
  - Preoperative clinic
  - Intraoperative anesthesia provider
  - Acute pain service
  - Chronic pain service/opioid transition clinic
- Surgical team
- Pharmacy
- Spiritual services
- Addiction medicine specialists
- Health psychology
- Physical medicine and rehabilitation
- Physical/occupational therapy
- Complementary medicine

Coordination with other services will facilitate long-term success.

physical and occupational therapy. Providers of integrative medicine (acupuncture, massage, hypnosis, etc) may also supply complementary therapies that aid in pain management [45].

The specifics of analgesic management prescribed by this inpatient team will vary depending on the patient, their personal history of pain symptoms and treatment modalities, and the surgical procedure. However, there are a number of treatment strategies that deserve general consideration. Multimodal analgesic approaches should be considered to decrease opioid administration and opioid-related side effects and to provide analgesia in patients for whom opioids are unlikely to be effective (Fig. 3) [48]. Nonpharmacologic efforts at pain management should also be encouraged as low-risk alternatives to opioid dose escalation (Box 2). These strategies might include distraction, meditation, mirror therapy, heat or ice, or transcutaneous electrical nerve stimulation devices. Finally, efforts to provide regional anesthesia should be maximized.

NONOPIOID PHARMACOLOGIC MECHANISMS TO TREAT PAIN

Regional anesthesia

Patients with a history of poorly controlled pain or opioid abuse may benefit from regional anesthetic procedures. Neuraxial and peripheral nerve blocks can block the transmission of painful stimuli and decrease the intensity of pain symptoms and opioid requirements for a variety of surgical

Preoperative	Intraoperative	Postoperative
• Acetaminophen PO	• Acetaminophen IV	• Acetaminophen PO/PR/IV
• NSAIDs PO	• NSAIDs IV	• NSAIDs PO/IV
• Gabapentinoids	• Ketamine	• Gabapentinoids
• Regional anesthesia	• Magnesium	• Ketamine
	• Alpha-2 agonists	• Lidocaine
	• Lidocaine	• Alpha-2 agonists
	• Dexamethasone	• Regional anesthesia
	• Esmolol	• Capsaicin
	• Regional anesthesia	• Opioid PO/IV PCA
	• Opioids	

Fig. 3. Pharmacologic approaches to perioperative management of the patient with medication-assisted treatment for substance abuse disorders. IV, intravenous; NSAIDs, nonsteroidal anti-inflammatory drugs; PO, orally; PR, per rectum.

procedures [49]. Decreases in acute postoperative pain may also result in a decreased frequency and severity of chronic pain symptoms. The introduction and adoption of fascial plane blocks, including erector spinae, retrolaminar, quadratous lumborum, pectoralis, and serratus anterior plane blocks, have allowed for an increase in the application of regional anesthesia procedures beyond what was traditionally available. Ultrasound guidance may improve

Box 2: Nonpharmacologic approaches to perioperative management of the patient with medication-assisted treatment for substance abuse disorders

Nonpharmacologic analgesic adjuncts for opioid tolerant patients

- Transcutaneous electrical nerve stimulation
- Heat/cold
- Acupuncture
- Massage
- Distraction
- Mindfulness/meditation
- Breathing exercises
- Mirror therapy
- Pastoral services
- Aromatherapy
- Hypnosis
- Music therapy
- Physical therapy

the safety and efficacy of regional anesthesia procedures and allow for even more widespread application [50]. Local anesthetic adjuncts (eg, clonidine and dexamethasone), liposomal formulations, or continuous catheter techniques should be considered to both prolong the duration of analgesia and decrease the incidence or severity of rebound pain. Surgical colleagues should be encouraged to provide surgical site administration of local anesthetic via either infiltration or continuous infusion techniques if a peripheral nerve block is contraindicated.

Intravenous lidocaine

The intravenous administration of lidocaine provides analgesia without the need for an invasive procedure. Intravenous infusions of lidocaine are proposed to be beneficial via sodium channel blockade-related analgesic and anti-inflammatory mechanisms that are yet to be well-defined [51]. Lidocaine may also directly act on the dorsal horn of the spinal cord to inhibit glutamate release [52], which may be why it is especially effective in treating neuropathic pain [53]. Although the literature is mixed with regard to efficacy, lidocaine infusions have demonstrated significant pain management benefits when used for select abdominal or thoracic procedures [54]. Other studies have demonstrated that perioperative lidocaine infusions are also associated with decreased hospital length of stay and earlier return of bowel function [55]. Patients with intravenous lidocaine infusions require close monitoring for the development of severe adverse neurologic or cardiac reactions and oftentimes infusions are discontinued at the time of discharge from the postanesthesia care unit secondary to limited monitoring capabilities on surgical floors [56]. Caution should be exercised in patients with a history of seizures, hepatic disease, or cardiac conduction abnormalities. Dosing should also be cautiously done in those with obesity or low muscle mass. See Table 2 for a potential dosing strategy.

Acetaminophen

Acetaminophen is a centrally acting analgesic that possesses weak anti-inflammatory properties. Preoperative oral acetaminophen administration represents an inexpensive mechanism to enhance perioperative analgesia. Rectal and intravenous routes of administration are also available, but suffer from either decreased provider–patient enthusiasm for route of administration or increased cost without significant benefits relative to oral administration [57]. In fact, a recent analysis has demonstrated that although both intravenous and oral acetaminophen decrease opioid consumption on postoperative day 1, oral acetaminophen decreases opioid consumption more effectively [58].

Ketamine

Perioperative ketamine use can decrease postoperative opioid requirements while simultaneously decreasing the development of opioid induced hyperalgesia via its NMDA receptor antagonism. Dextromethorphan and amantadine have also been administered to provide NMDA receptor antagonism, but are much less frequently used in a clinical setting [59]. In 1 study of

Table 2
Potential dosing strategies for various analgesics that can be used as part of a multimodal approach

Medication	Potential dosing strategy	Route of administration
Acetaminophen	1000 mg before surgery QID dosing postoperatively	PO, PR, IV
Lidocaine	1–2 mg/kg bolus at induction 1–2 mg/kg/h infusion	IV
Ketamine	0.25–0.5 mg/kg IV bolus at induction 2–10 μg/kg/min intraoperatively 10–12 mg/h postoperatively	IV
Gabapentin	600 mg before surgery 600 mg TID postoperatively	PO
NSAIDs	Ketorolac: 15–30 mg QID Celecoxib: 200 mg QD	Ketorolac: IV Celecoxib: PO
Alpha-2 agonists	Dexmedetomidine: 1 μg/kg load over 10 min with 0.2–1.4 μg/kg/h infusion Clonidine: 200 μg/d	Dexmedetomidine: IV Clonidine: PO or TD
Magnesium	250 mg bolus at induction 500 mg/h infusion	IV
Esmolol	0.5–1 mg/kg at induction 5–50 μg/kg/min infusion	IV
Dexamethasone	0.1 mg/kg at induction	IV

Abbreviations: IM, intramuscular; IV, intravenous; NSAIDs, nonsteroidal anti-inflammatory drugs; PO, orally; PR, per rectum; QD, daily; QID, 4 times per day; TD, transdermal; TID, 3 times per day.

opioid-tolerant patients undergoing spine surgery, intraoperative ketamine administration demonstrated long-lasting pain management and opioid sparing effects that were sustained at 6 weeks after surgery [60]. Other studies have demonstrated that decreases in sedation and pain scores after ketamine administration persisted at 6 months after surgical procedures [61]. Ketamine therapy is well-tolerated, but rare hallucinations, liver function test elevations, sympathetic stimulation, or increases in intracranial pressure may limit the ability to safely prescribe this agent in select patients [62]. Ketamine infusion therapy is commonly safely administered on a general care floor, but local institutional policies may dictate a higher level of care and monitoring. See Table 2 for a potential dosing strategy.

Dexamethasone

Dexamethasone at doses of 0.1 to 0.2 mg/kg are effective at decreasing postoperative pain and opioid administration [63,64]. Perineural administration of dexamethasone may also provide prolongation of regional anesthesia techniques [65]. See Table 2 for a potential dosing strategy.

Esmolol

Recent evidence suggests that intraoperative esmolol infusions can decrease intraoperative opioid administration, postanesthesia care unit pain, and postanesthesia care unit opioid requirements. The mechanism of pain reduction associated with esmolol infusions is unclear but may be related to diminishing the impact of opioid induced hyperalgesia by limiting intraoperative opioid administration [66]. See Table 2 for a potential dosing strategy.

Gabapentin

Gabapentinoids (gabapentin and pregabalin) bind to an auxiliary subunit of voltage-dependent calcium channels, which in turn inhibit the release of excitatory neurotransmitters. The gabapentinoids have been successfully used to decrease both acute postsurgical and chronic postoperative pain [67,68]. Other studies have also demonstrated diminished postoperative opioid requirements with perioperative gabapentin [69]. The ideal dosing regimen has not yet been well-established, but reductions in dosing should generally be considered in the elderly and those with significant renal impairment. Dosing may be limited by the development of significant nausea or sedation. In the setting of acute pain, doses of gabapentinoids can generally be discontinued after 2 weeks of therapy [70]. See Table 2 for a potential dosing strategy.

Alpha-2 agonists

In the realm of pain management, alpha-2 agonists (clonidine and dexmedetomidine) act at the dorsal horn of the spinal cord to dampen the transmission of painful impulses. Use may be limited by the development of side effects, including sedation, bradycardia, and hypotension. Parenteral forms are available for both clonidine and dexmedetomidine, but clonidine is also available as a tablet, patch, or transdermal cream. This may increase the applicability and tolerance of this agent. Finally, perineural alpha-2 agonists have also been used to provide prolongation of regional anesthesia techniques [71]. See Table 2 for a potential dosing strategy.

Magnesium

Magnesium exerts its analgesic effect via antagonism at NMDA and calcium channel receptors. A 2013 meta-analysis demonstrated decreased pain and opioid requirements for 24 hours after surgery [72]. Dosing reductions or omission should be considered in patients with significant renal failure because accumulations may occur. In addition, neuromuscular blockade should be monitored closely for prolongation in the setting of magnesium supplementation. See Table 2 for a potential dosing strategy.

Nonsteroidal anti-inflammatory drugs

Nonsteroidal anti-inflammatory drugs represent an additional inexpensive analgesic modality that is, available for administration via either the oral or intravenous route. Nonsteroidal anti-inflammatory drugs function via inhibition of the cyclooxygenase enzyme. Concern over the potential for nonsteroidal anti-inflammatory drugs to inhibit platelet aggregation or impact renal function may limit the ability to administer these agents in the perioperative setting. However, the risk of increased surgical or gastrointestinal bleeding is not significantly affected with the postoperative administration of ketorolac, an intravenous cyclooxygenase-1 inhibitor [73,74]. Ketorolac dosing should be limited to

5 days over concerns related to adverse gastrointestinal or renal effects. Cyclooxygenase-2 inhibitors, such as celecoxib, may be less likely to result in clinically significant postsurgical bleeding and may therefore be better tolerated in certain clinical scenarios. However, patients with significant cardiac abnormalities (heart failure or revascularization) may not be appropriate candidates for nonsteroidal anti-inflammatory drug therapy because they may have an increased risk of thrombotic events, including myocardial infarction and stroke. See Table 2 for a potential dosing strategy.

Opioids

For patients with a history of opioid dependency or currently prescribed maintenance therapy with agents intended to curb opioid abuse, an opioid-free anesthetic, if possible, may be the preferred analgesic technique. To accomplish this goal, patients must be a motivated component of the decision-making process and regional and multimodal analgesic administration must be maximized. If opioid therapy cannot be avoided, consideration should be given to using multimodal intraoperative analgesic regimens that avoid rapid-acting or ever-escalating doses of intraoperative opioids that can result in acute tolerance and increased postoperative dosing requirements [75]. Baseline opioid therapy, partial opioid agonists, or opioid antagonists may make postoperative opioid dosing requirements quite high. These patients may therefore be at increased risk for postoperative respiratory depression and should be closely monitored [76]. Alternatively, loading patients with methadone intraoperatively has been shown to decrease the need for postoperative opioids, decrease patient-reported pain scores, and improve overall patient satisfaction [25]. Opioid rotations may be beneficial to some patients, but this practice should be closely directed by an inpatient pain service. Finally, in patients with a history of substance abuse, consideration should be given to prescribing an appropriate discharge analgesic regimen that decreases the likelihood of abuse. For example, newer formulations of extended-release oxycodone (eg, Xtampza ER and REMOXY ER) may decrease the risk of abuse or diversion by lessening the impact of drug crushing and injection [77,78]. Any changes to the home-going analgesic regimen should be closely communicated to the patient's outpatient opioid prescriber and consideration should be given to coordinating care with an opioid transition clinic. Opioid prescriptions for these patients should be for a limited time period, be limited in dose, and refills should not be allowed without reevaluation.

SUMMARY

There are many patients in treatment for opioid abuse disorders and this number will likely continue to increase. Appropriately treating these patients in the perioperative period requires a thoughtful and multidisciplinary approach that considers the patient's individual pain management history, history of opioid-related use or abuse, and history of effective analgesic management therapies. Management of these patients begins well before the day of surgery and not simply in the postoperative period. Although the management of these patients may be associated with significant difficulties, the opportunity to provide effective and compassionate pain management will be deeply appreciated by the patient, their family, and your surgical colleagues. Ultimately, the management of these complex patients represents a phenomenal opportunity for anesthesiologists to distinguish themselves as experts in pain management and essential components of the entire arc of the perioperative process.

References

[1] Koepke EJ, Manning EL, Miller TE, et al. The rising tide of opioid use and abuse: the role of the anesthesiologist. Perioper Med (Lond) 2018;7:16.

[2] CDC Centers for Disease Control and Prevention. Opioid overdose – drug overdose deaths. Available at: https://www.cdc.gov/drugoverdose/data/statedeaths.html. Accessed June 26, 2019.

[3] National Institute on Drug Abuse. Opioid overdose crisis. Available at: https://www.drugabuse.gov/drugs-abuse/opioids/opioid-overdose-crisis#one. Accessed June 26, 2019.

[4] Hedegaard H, Minino AM, Warner M. Drug overdose deaths in the United States, 1999-2017. NCHS Data Brief 2018;329:1–8. Available at: https://www.cdc.gov/nchs/data/databriefs/db329-h.pdf. Accessed June 26, 2019.

[5] Murphy SL, Xu JQ, Kochanek KD, et al. Mortality in the United States, 2017. NCHS Data Brief 2018;328:1–8. Available at: https://www.cdc.gov/nchs/products/databriefs/db328.htm. Accessed June 26, 2019.

[6] Florence CS, Zhou C, Luo F, et al. The economic burden of prescription opioid overdose, abuse, and dependence in the United States, 2013. Med Care 2016;54:901–6.

[7] Peppin JF. The marginalization of chronic pain patients on chronic opioid therapy. Pain Physician 2009;12:493–8.

[8] Kharasch ED, Brunt LM. Perioperative opioids and public health. Anesthesiology 2016;124:960–5.

[9] Kehlet H, Jensen TS, Woolf CJ. Persistent postsurgical pain: risk factors and prevention. Lancet 2006;367:1618–25.

[10] Waljee JF, Cron DC, Steiger RM, et al. Effect of preoperative opioid exposure on healthcare utilization and expenditures following elective abdominal surgery. Ann Surg 2017;265: 715–21.

[11] Center for Substance Abuse Treatment. Clinical guidelines for the use of buprenorphine in the treatment of opioid addiction. Treatment Improvement Protocol (TIP) Series, vol. 20. Rockville (MD): Substance Abuse and Mental Health Services Administration; 2004.

[12] Dahan A, Yassen A, Romberg R, et al. Buprenorphine induces ceiling in respiratory depression but not in analgesia. Br J Anaesth 2006;96(5):627–32.

[13] Dahan A. Opioid-induced respiratory effects: new data on buprenorphine. Palliat Med 2006;20(Suppl 1):s3–8.

[14] Drug bank: buprenorphine. 2019. Available at: https://www.drugbank.ca/drugs/DB00921. Accessed March 27, 2019.

[15] Volpe DA, McMahon Tobin GA, Mellon RD, et al. Uniform assessment and ranking of opioid mu receptor binding constants for selected opioid drugs. Regul Toxicol Pharmacol 2011;59(3):385–90.

[16] Jones RG, Groeger LV, Ornstein C. Prescriber checkup. 2019. Available at: https://projects.propublica.org/checkup/. Accessed April 1, 2019.

[17] Quaye AN, Zhang Y. Perioperative management of buprenorphine: solving the conundrum. Pain Med 2018;20(7):1–14.

[18] Goel A, Azargive S, Lamba W, et al. The perioperative patient on buprenorphine: a systematic review of perioperative management strategies and patient outcomes. Can J Anaesth 2019;66(2):201–17.

[19] Macintyre PE, Russell RA, Usher KA, et al. Pain relief and opioid requirements in the first 24 hours after surgery in patients taking buprenorphine and methadone opioid substitution therapy. Anaesth Intensive Care 2013;41(2):222–30.
[20] Lemke A, Ottestad E, Schmiesing C. Patients maintained on buprenorphine for opioid use disorder should continue buprenorphine through the perioperative period. Pain Med 2019;20(3):425–8.
[21] Anderson TA, Quaye ANA, Ward EN, et al. To stop or not, that is the question: acute pain management for the patient on chronic buprenorphine. Anesthesiology 2017;126(6): 1180–6.
[22] Kampman K, Jarvis M. ASAM National practice guideline for the use of medications in the treatment of addiction involving opioid use. J Addict Med 2015;9(5):358–67.
[23] Sordo L, Barrio G, Bravo MJ, et al. Mortality risk during and after opioid substitution treatment: systematic review and meta-analysis of cohort studies. BMJ 2017;357:j1550.
[24] Bentzley BS, Barth KS, Back SE, et al. Discontinuation of buprenorphine maintenance therapy: perspectives and outcomes. J Subst Abuse Treat 2015;52:48–57.
[25] Murphy GS, Szokol JW, Avram MJ, et al. Clinical effectiveness and safety of intraoperative methadone in patients undergoing posterior spinal fusion surgery: a randomized, double-blinded, controlled trial. Anesthesiology 2017;126(5):822–33.
[26] Kharasch ED. Intraoperative methadone: rediscovery, reappraisal, and reinvigoration? Anesth Analg 2011;112(1):13–6.
[27] Harrison TK, Kornfeld H, Aggarwal AK, et al. Perioperative considerations for the patient with opioid use disorder on buprenorphine, methadone, or naltrexone maintenance therapy. Anesthesiology Clin 2018;36:345–59.
[28] Peng PWH, Tumber PS, Gourlay D. Review article: perioperative pain management of patients on methadone therapy. Can J Anaesth 2005;15(5):513–23.
[29] Methadone. Lexicomp. Riverwoods (IL): Wolters Kluwer Health, Inc. Available at: http://online.lexi.com. Accessed February 22, 2018.
[30] Fishman SM, Wilsey B, Mahajan G, et al. Methadone reincarnated: novel clinical applications with related concerns. Pain Med 2002;3(4):339–48.
[31] Noble F, Marie N. Management of opioid addiction with opioid substitution treatments: beyond methadone and buprenorphine. Front Psychiatry 2019;9(742):1–8.
[32] McCance-Katz EF, Sullivan L, Nallani S. Drug interactions of clinical importance among the opioids, methadone and buprenorphine and other frequently prescribed medications: a review. Am J Addict 2010;19(1):4–16.
[33] ReVia®. In: Drugs@FDA: FDA approved drug products. Available at: https://www.accessdata.fda.gov/drugsatfda_docs/label/2013/018932s017lbl.pdf. Accessed March 7, 2019.
[34] Volkow ND. Medications for opioid use disorder: bridging the gap in care. Lancet 2018;391:285–7.
[35] Tanum L, Solli KK, Latif Z, et al. Effectiveness of injectable extended-release naltrexone vs daily buprenorphine-naloxone for opioid dependence: a randomized clinical noninferiority trial. JAMA Psychiatry 2017;74(12):1197–205.
[36] Lee JD, Nunes EV, Novo P, et al. Comparative effectiveness of extended-release naltrexone versus buprenorphine-naloxone for opioid relapse prevention (X:BOT): a multicentre, open-label, randomised controlled trial. Lancet 2018;391(10118):309–18.
[37] Krupitsky E, Nunes EV, Ling W, et al. Injectable extended-release naltrexone for opioid dependence: a double-blind, placebo-controlled, multicentre randomised trial. Lancet 2011;377:1506–13.
[38] Morgan JR, Schackman BR, Leff JA, et al. Injectable naltrexone, oral naltrexone, and buprenorphine utilization and discontinuation among individuals treated for opioid use disorder in a United States commercially insured population. J Subst Abuse Treat 2018;85:90–6.

[39] Patten DK, Schultz BG, Berlau DJ. The safety and efficacy of low-dose naltrexone in the management of chronic pain and inflammation in multiple sclerosis, fibromyalgia, Crohn's disease, and other chronic pain disorders. Pharmacotherapy 2018;38(3):382–9.
[40] Trofimovitch D, Baumrucker SJ. Pharmacology update: low-dose naltrexone as a possible nonopioid modality for some chronic, nonmalignant pain syndromes. Am J Hosp Palliat Med 2019;36(10).
[41] Naltrexone. Lexicomp. Riverwoods (IL): Wolters Kluwer Health, Inc. Available at: http://online.lexi.com. Accessed February 22, 2018.
[42] Minozzi S, Amato L, Vecchi S, et al. Oral naltrexone maintenance treatment for opioid dependence. Cochrane Database Syst Rev 2011;(4):CD001333.
[43] Coluzzi F, Bifulco F, Cuomo A, et al. The challenge of perioperative pain management in opioid-tolerant patients. Ther Clin Risk Manag 2017;13:1163–73.
[44] Zaccagnino MF, Bader AM, Sang CN, et al. The perioperative surgical home: a new role for the acute pain service. Anesth Analg 2017;125:1394–402.
[45] Hanna MN, Speed TJ, Shechter R, et al. An innovative perioperative pain program for chronic opioid users: an academic medical center's response to the opioid crisis. Am J Med Qual 2019;34:5–13.
[46] Vetter TR, Kain ZN. Role of the perioperative surgical home in optimizing the perioperative use of opioids. Anesth Analg 2017;125:1653–7.
[47] Khan TW, Manion S. Perioperative surgical home for the patient with chronic pain. Anesthesiology Clin 2018;36:281–94.
[48] Kehlet H, Dahl JB. The value of "multimodal" or "balanced analgesia" in postoperative pain treatment. Anesth Analg 1993;77:1048–56.
[49] Donauer K, Bomberg H, Wagenpfeil S, et al. Regional vs. general anesthesia for total knee and hip replacement: an analysis of postoperative pain perception from the international PAIN OUT registry. Pain Pract 2018;18(8):1036–47.
[50] Barrington MJ, Uda Y. Did ultrasound fulfill the promise of safety in regional anesthesia? Curr Opin Anaesthesiol 2018;31(5):649–55.
[51] Rogers M, Tang L, Madge DJ, et al. The role of sodium channels in neuropathic pain. Semin Cell Dev Biol 2006;17:571–81.
[52] Kurabe M, Furue H, Kohno T. Intravenous administration of lidocaine directly acts on spinal dorsal horn and produces analgesic effect: an in vivo patch-clamp analysis. Sci Rep 2016;6:26253.
[53] Kandil E, Melikman E, Adinoff B. Lidocaine infusion: a promising therapeutic approach for chronic pain. J Anesth Clin Res 2017;8(1):697.
[54] Dunn LK, Durieux ME. Perioperative use of intravenous lidocaine. Anesthesiology 2017;126:729–37.
[55] Vigneault L, Turgeon AF, Cote D, et al. Perioperative intravenous lidocaine infusion for postoperative pain control: a meta-analysis of randomized controlled trials. Can J Anaesth 2011;58(1):22–37.
[56] Eipe N, Gupta S, Penning J. Intravenous lidocaine for acute pain: an evidence-based clinical update. BJA Educ 2016;16:292–8.
[57] Jibril F, Sharaby S, Mohamed A, et al. Intravenous versus oral acetaminophen for pain: systematic review of current evidence to support clinical decision-making. Can J Hosp Pharm 2015;68:238–47.
[58] Wasserman I, Poeran J, Zubizaretta N, et al. Impact of intravenous acetaminophen on perioperative opioid utilization and outcomes in open colectomies: a claims database analysis. Anesthesiology 2018;129(1):77–88.
[59] Carrol IR, Angst MS, Clark JD. Management of perioperative pain in patients chronically consuming opioids. Reg Anesth Pain Med 2004;29:576–91.
[60] Loftus RW, Yeager MP, Clark JA, et al. Intraoperative ketamine reduces perioperative opioid consumption in opiate-dependent patients with chronic back pain undergoing back surgery. Anesthesiology 2010;113(3):639–46.

[61] Neilsen R, Fomsgaard JS, Siegel H, et al. Intraoperative ketamine reduces immediate postoperative opioid consumption after spinal fusion surgery in chronic pain patients with opioid dependency: a randomized, blinded trial. Pain 2017;158:463–70.
[62] Schwenk ES, Goldberg SF, Patel RD, et al. Adverse drug effects and preoperative medication factors related to low-dose ketamine infusions. Reg Anesth Pain Med 2016;41:482–7.
[63] De Oliveira GS Jr, Almeida MD, Benzon HT, et al. Perioperative single dose systemic dexamethasone for postoperative pain. Anesthesiology 2011;115(3):575–88.
[64] Meng J, Li L. The efficiency and safety of dexamethasone for pain control in total joint arthroplasty: a meta-analysis of controlled trials. Medicine 2017;96(24):e7126.
[65] Zhang D, Zhou C, Wei D, et al. Dexamethasone added to local anesthetics in ultrasound-guided transversus abdominis plain (TAP) block for analgesia after abdominal surgery: a systematic review and meta-analysis of randomized controlled trials. PLoS One 2019;14(1):e0209646.
[66] Gelineau AM, King MR, Ladha KS, et al. Intraoperative esmolol as an adjunct for perioperative opioid and postoperative pain reduction: a systemic review, meta-analysis, and meta-regression. Anesth Analg 2018;126(3):1035–49.
[67] Hurley RW, Cohen SP, Williams KA, et al. The analgesic effects of perioperative gabapentin on postoperative pain: a meta-analysis. Reg Anesth Pain Med 2006;31:237–47.
[68] Zhang J, Ho KY, Wang Y. Efficacy of pregabalin in acute postoperative pain: a meta-analysis. Br J Anaesth 2011;106(4):454–62.
[69] Wick EC, Association AM, Grant MC, et al. Postoperative multimodal analgesia pain management with nonopioid analgesics and techniques. JAMA Surg 2017;152(7):691.
[70] Thomas DA, Boominathan P, Goswami J, et al. Perioperative management of patients with addiction to opioid and non-opioid medications. Curr Pain Headache Rep 2018;22:52.
[71] Pöpping DM, Elia N, Marret E, et al. Clonidine as an adjuvant to local anesthetics for peripheral nerve and plexus blocks: a meta-analysis of randomized trials. Anesthesiology 2009;111:406–15.
[72] Albrecht E, Kirkham KR, Liu SS, et al. Peri-operative intravenous administration of magnesium sulfate and postoperative pain: a meta-analysis. Anaesthesia 2013;68:79–90.
[73] Gobble RM, Hoang HLT, Kachniarz B, et al. Ketorolac does not increase perioperative bleeding: a meta-analysis of randomized controlled trials. Plast Reconstr Surg 2014;133(3):741–55.
[74] De Oliveira GS Jr, Agarwal D, Benzon HT. Perioperative single dose ketorolac to prevent postoperative pain: a meta-analysis of randomized trials. Anesth Analg 2012;114(2):424–33.
[75] Chia YY, Liu K, Wang JJ, et al. Intraoperative high dose fentanyl induces postoperative fentanyl tolerance. Can J Anaesth 1999;46:872–7.
[76] Hayhurst CK, Durieux ME. Differential opioid tolerance and opioid-induced hyperalgesia: a clinical reality. Anesthesiology 2016;124:483–8.
[77] Meske D, Kopecky EA, Passik S, et al. Evaluation of the oral human abuse potential of Oxycodone DETERx® formulation (Xtampsa® ER). J Opioid Manag 2018;14(5):359–72.
[78] Kucera SA, Zamloot MS, Crowley MM, et al. Abuse-deterrent properties of REMOXY® ER, a high-viscosity extended-release oxycodone formulation. J Opioid Manag 2018;4(6):429–36.

Advances in Anesthesia 37 (2019) 87–110

ADVANCES IN ANESTHESIA

Tranexamic Acid in the Perioperative Period

Yes, No, Maybe?

Justin E. Richards, MD[a], Ron E. Samet, MD[a], A. Kennedy Koerner, MD[b], Thomas E. Grissom, MD, MSIS, FCCM[a,*]

[a]Department of Anesthesiology, University of Maryland School of Medicine, R Adams Cowley Shock Trauma Center, 22 South Greene Street, Suite T1R77, Baltimore, MD 21201, USA; [b]Department of Anesthesiology, University of Maryland School of Medicine, Center for the Sustainment of Trauma and Readiness Skills (CSTARS)-Baltimore, R Adams Cowley Shock Trauma Center, 22 South Greene Street, Suite T1R77, Baltimore, MD 21201, USA

Keywords

• Trauma • Tranexamic acid • Hemorrhagic shock • Cardiac surgery • Resuscitation • Obstetric hemorrhage

Key points

- Antifibrinolytics have a role in the management of acute bleeding states as part of a blood conservation strategy.
- Early tranexamic acid administration has been shown to decrease blood loss and death from hemorrhage for trauma and postpartum hemorrhage without an increase in thromboembolic events.
- Although using tranexamic acid during orthotopic liver transplantation results in lower blood loss, its use is guided by viscoelastic hemostatic assay monitoring rather than an empiric approach in most programs.
- Routine use of tranexamic acid is common in major orthopedic spine, joint replacement, and trauma surgery.

Continued

Note: All authors played a role in the preparation of the article, figures, and tables. All authors attest to having approved the final article.

Funding Source: None.

Conflicts of Interest: The authors have identified no conflicts of interest.

*Corresponding author. *E-mail address:* tgrissom@som.umaryland.edu

https://doi.org/10.1016/j.aan.2019.08.009
0737-6146/19/

Continued

- Tranexamic acid or other antifibrinolytics for cardiac surgery results in less blood loss, fewer transfusions, and less need for reoperation, although the optimal dosing strategy has not been established.

INTRODUCTION

Fibrinolysis is a physiologic element of hemostasis that works to regulate clot formation through enzymatic breakdown of fibrin blood clots. Like the coagulation cascade, fibrinolysis is closely controlled by a series of cofactors, inhibitors, and receptors. In the perioperative period, tissue injury associated with trauma or surgery, blood contact with large nonendothelial surfaces such as cardiopulmonary bypass circuits, or ischemia and reperfusion may produce excessive fibrinolysis, contributing to worsened coagulopathy or bleeding. As a result, significant evidence in the perioperative setting has supported the efficacy of antifibrinolytic agents to reduce blood loss and decrease allogeneic blood administration without an increase in adverse clinical outcomes. Of all the antifibrinolytic agents, tranexamic acid (TXA) is currently the most extensively studied.

Introduced in the 1960s, the fibrinolytic inhibitor TXA has been used in a number of clinical situations to decrease bleeding and associated complications. Despite studies dating back to the late 1960s [1,2], the use of TXA only slowly gained traction in the routine management of perioperative bleeding until the early 2000s. Over the last 20 years, the clinical use of TXA has expanded significantly as evidenced by the amount of research and number of publications focusing on its use in a broad range of clinical applications (Fig. 1). In this review, we briefly look at the history and pharmacology of TXA before summarizing the most recent clinical experience and recommendations.

BACKGROUND

TXA has gained increased attention in the last few decades as a potent antifibrinolytic agent that inhibits clot breakdown and decreases bleeding, transfusion requirements, and mortality in various clinical settings. Synthesized in the 1960s in response to the high rate of postpartum hemorrhage (PPH) and associated mortality, trans-4-aminomethyl-cyclohexanecarboxylic acid, renamed TXA, is a more potent modification of the first antifibrinolytic discovered, epsilon-aminocaproic acid (EACA) [3]. Although EACA is a powerful inhibitor of plasminogen, large doses are required to achieve a clinical effect. The search for a more potent agent led to the discovery of TXA in both Japan and Sweden during the same time period [4].

Slow to adopt in the obstetric population, the drug became popular for patients with hereditary bleeding disorders for whom menorrhagia, frequent spontaneous nose bleeds, or dental procedures could be life threatening. More recently, its use has expanded to treat or prevent excessive blood loss

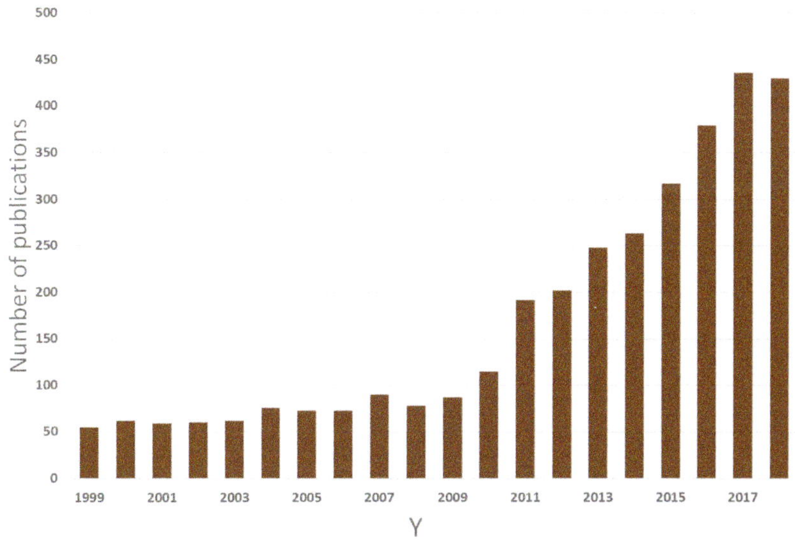

Fig. 1. Results from PubMed for search term TXA from medical subject headings, title, and abstract for 1999 to 2018.

from trauma and major surgery, including cardiac, orthopedic, and hepatic procedures. With a strong record as an effective and safe medicine, TXA has earned its place on the World Health Organization List of Essential Medicines as an important drug needed in every health system [5].

Several landmark studies have likely led to the expanded use of TXA in clinical practice. The Clinical Randomization of an Antifibrinolytic in Significant Hemorrhage 2 (CRASH-2) trial enrolled more than 20,000 patients in 274 hospitals and found an overall decrease in all-cause mortality and risk of death owing to bleeding when TXA was administered to acutely bleeding patients, without evidence of increased fatal or nonfatal vascular occlusive events [6]. Similarly, the World Maternal Antifibrinolytic (WOMAN) trial that recently evaluated the efficacy of TXA for prevention of death owing to PPH after a vaginal birth or caesarian section highlighted the potential for TXA in a large, at-risk population enrolling more than 20,000 women in this multisite, international study [7]. The collaborators found similar significant decreases in maternal death owing to bleeding in the TXA group with no appreciable differences in thromboembolic events between the treatment and placebo groups. Early treatment in the obstetric population was also advised and fortified the inclusion of TXA in the World Health Organization treatment guidelines for primary PPH [8]. Because of these large studies and other work, including patients undergoing cardiac, orthopedic, and hepatic surgery, TXA administration has become more commonplace, especially in locations with limited blood transfusion capabilities.

Currently, the most common antifibrinolytic agents in use are EACA and TXA. A third agent, aprotinin, was withdrawn from the market in 2007 owing to safety concerns noted in several studies, suggesting an increased risk of death and renal dysfunction in patients undergoing cardiac surgery [9,10]. Since its withdrawal from the market, several methodologic concerns have been raised regarding the adverse outcomes from earlier trials resulting in its reintroduction in Canada [11] and in Europe [12] for isolated coronary bypass surgery. More recent work, however, continues to suggest that aprotinin may carry additional risk leading to ongoing concerns regarding the relative risk-benefit assessment for its use [13]. The remainder of this update focuses on TXA because it continues to be the most commonly used antifibrinolytic agent.

PHARMACOLOGY

Pharmacodynamics

The process of fibrinolysis requires inactive plasminogen to bind to fibrin clot via lysine binding domains. Subsequently, plasminogen becomes activated by tissue plasminogen activator (tPA) or the cell receptor-bound urokinase plasminogen activator, thereby cleaving fibrin-bound plasminogen to its active protease form, plasmin (Fig. 2) [14]. Once activated, plasmin (fibrinolysin) works to degrade fibrin clot, fibrinogen, and other plasma proteins, including the procoagulant factors V and VIII. This process leads to limited clot formation under normal conditions of hemostasis. TXA functions as a synthetic analog of

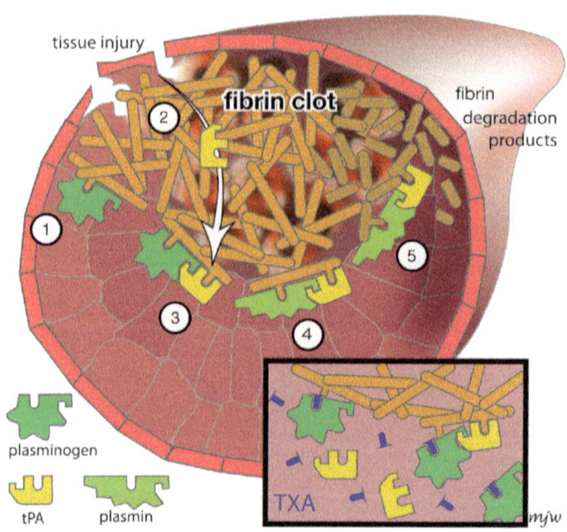

Fig. 2. Intravascular fibrinolysis and the antifibrinolytic mechanism of action of TXA. (1) Plasminogen binds to fibrin in a clot via lysine receptors on plasminogen yet remains inactive in lysing the clot. (2) Tissue injury initiates a release of tPA from endothelial cells. (3) tPA binds to fibrin and to plasminogen on the fibrin clot. (4) tPA binding leads to a conformational change in the bound plasminogen to its active form, plasmin. (5) Plasmin cleaves the fibrin molecules and the clot dissolves into fibrin degradation products. TXA, a lysine analogue, reversibly binds to the plasminogen lysine receptors and thereby blocks plasminogen from binding to fibrin. Because tPA can only activate fibrin-bound plasminogen, subsequent plasmin activation is impaired with resultant fibrinolysis inhibition.

the amino acid lysine to competitively inhibit plasminogen from binding to fibrin and consequently indirectly inhibits plasmin formation. Additionally, a high concentration of TXA can directly inhibit plasmin activity, albeit at a low affinity and of questionable clinical significance. Some recent studies demonstrate that TXA can also attenuate endogenous urokinase plasminogen activator activity independent of plasminogen activation [14]. Interestingly, in acute trauma, upregulations of plasma urokinase plasminogen activator 3 hours or more postinjury makes TXA less efficacious as an antifibrinolytic and may explain the lack of efficacy when administered more than 3 hours after injury [15].

It is also worth noting that TXA has been used in hereditary angioedema to prevent attacks via reduction of plasmin-induced activation of the first complement protein, C1. As such, activation of the complement system and immune cells is diminished and can limit symptoms of angioedema [16]. Side effects have been reported to include gastrointestinal upset, joint and muscle pain, headache, and allergic symptomology. Importantly, TXA inadvertently injected into the spinal space, most commonly owing to administration errors, has led to catastrophic cardiovascular and neurologic complications with an almost 50% fatality rate in a recent review [17].

Pharmacokinetics

TXA is available in intravenous (IV), oral, and topical formulations. Administration via IV injection of 10 mg/kg in healthy volunteers achieved peak plasma concentrations within 1 hour of administration with a half-life of approximately 80 minutes, whereas oral intake of 10 to 15 mg/kg took 3 hours to achieve peak concentration [18]. Near 100% fibrinolytic inhibition (in vitro) is observed with plasma concentrations of 100 mg/L, although an 80% inhibition is likely satisfactory with plasma concentrations of 10 mg/L [19]. TXA diffuses into joint and synovial membranes and appears in extremely dilute concentrations in fetal circulation and breast milk with no known teratogenic effects [20–22]. Clearance of TXA occurs via glomerular filtration with 30% excreted in the first hour and 90% after 24 hours in healthy individuals. For those with renal impairment, dosage modifications must be made to avoid toxic accumulation [23]. Finally, topical administration has been studied and seems to be equally efficacious compared with IV TXA in many clinical settings [24].

CLINICAL CONSIDERATIONS WITH TRANEXAMIC ACID

Obstetrics

Globally, obstetric hemorrhage remains the leading cause of maternal mortality, particularly in low- and middle-income countries [25]. As noted, the original development of TXA was largely driven by a desire to address the problem of PPH. Despite this initial focus, work before the WOMAN trial [7] published in 2017 provided little information to guide the use of TXA in the management of obstetric hemorrhage [26–28]. Several of these reviews and meta-analyses acknowledged a potential role for TXA; however, the heterogeneity of the data and a focus on low-risk patients undergoing cesarean section called for further work to be done in a higher risk population with ongoing hemorrhage. Before the WOMAN trial, there was only a single, small, randomized, controlled trial of TXA for PPH that reported a reduction in blood loss and maternal morbidity [29]. Ducloy-Bouthers and colleagues [29] found that high -dose TXA (4 g over 1 hour followed by 1 g/h over 6 hour) in combination with traditional uterotonics was associated with a slight decrease in blood loss as well as a decrease in transfusion requirements and progression to severe PPH. The study was underpowered to address the question of mortality, and the exceedingly high dose was in excess of that used outside of cardiac surgery at the time.

Given the significant impact of hemorrhage on maternal mortality, the WOMAN trial was a natural follow-on to the CRASH-2 trial, where early TXA use was associated with less death owing to hemorrhage. Like the CRASH-2 trial, a broad range of study sites was included from low- to high-resource countries given the higher prevalence of maternal death owing to hemorrhage in less resource intensive health care settings. The WOMAN trial was originally designed to enroll 15,000 patients with a combined primary end point of all-cause mortality or hysterectomy with a 90% power to detect a 25% relative decrease. Clinicians were able to enroll patients when they were uncertain about whether to use TXA in a woman with PPH, at which time the patient was randomly assigned to receive TXA or placebo in a blinded, controlled fashion. Although the definition of PPH was defined as a clinically estimated blood loss of more than 500 mL for a vaginal delivery and more than 1000 mL for a cesarean delivery, the investigators also allowed inclusion for any patient felt to have enough blood loss to compromise hemodynamic status. The patients enrolled into the TXA arm of the study received 1 g of TXA (100 mg/mL) at a rate of 10 mg/min with the ability to administer a repeat does if the bleeding persisted beyond 30 minutes or recurred within 24 hours of delivery.

During the data collection period, the investigators found that the decision to proceed to hysterectomy was frequently made at the same time as randomization. Because this factor would bias the composite outcome used in their initial power calculations, they revised the primary outcome to all-cause mortality, which increased their enrollment target to 20,000. This change was accomplished before unblinding of the data and performance of any group analyses, so it was assumed this would have minimum impact on the results. Ultimately, they enrolled 20,060 women with randomization to TXA (n = 10,051) or placebo (n = 10,009) with 20,002 (99.7%) receiving the first dose of assigned study treatment. The final dataset for outcome analysis included 20,201 women. The investigators did not find a difference in all-cause mortality (227 [2.3%] in the TXA group vs 256 [2.6%] in the placebo group; relative risk [RR], 0.88; 95% confidence interval [CI], 0.74–1.05; $P = .16$) although death owing to hemorrhage was reduced in the TXA group (155 [1.5%] vs 191 [1.9%]; RR, 0.81; 95% CI, 0.65–1.00; $P = .045$). The impact of TXA on mortality was even greater when administered within 3 hours of giving birth (89 [1.2%] in the TXA group vs 127 [1.7%] in the placebo group; RR, 0.69; 95% CI, 0.52–0.91; $P = .008$). Additionally, they found a decrease in the need for laparotomy to control hemorrhage (82 [0.8%] in the TXA group vs 127 [1.3%] in the placebo group; RR, 0.64; 95% CI, 0.49–0.85; $P = .02$). The number needed to treat to prevent 1 death from bleeding was between 200 and 250 depending on time of administration. Of primary interest to many reviewers, the use of TXA was not associated with an increased incidence of thromboembolic events or other significant complications, including postpartum seizures.

As expected in a study of this nature, some interpretation of the results is required to assess the potential role of TXA in the management of PPH. One of the criticisms regards the role of TXA in mature comprehensive programs for PPH. Similar to questions raised in the CRASH-2 trial when comparing trauma management in low- and middle-resource countries with ones with a more mature trauma system, the benefits of TXA may not be as apparent in a setting with more resources and a robust response to clinical deterioration. The American College of Obstetricians and Gynecologists takes this view in their recommendation that TXA be used as a second line agent in cases of PPH not responsive to first-line agents, such as uterotonics [30]. In contrast, the World Health Organization has recommended that TXA be used in all cases of PPH concomitantly with uterotonics as a first-line agent, because 99% of all maternal deaths occur in low- and middle-income countries [8]. Assuming resources are available, it would seem reasonable to recommend TXA administration in the setting of severe PPH or when severe hemorrhage is anticipated based on maternal factors.

Currently, there is no consensus on the prophylactic use of TXA in the obstetric setting, but several upcoming studies will address this question. Additional data should be available in the next 2 years with work being done by the Eunice Kennedy Shriver National Institute of Child Health and Human Development examining the effect of prophylactic TXA before cesarean section in the United States in a double-blind, placebo-controlled trial [31]. This study is ongoing with a targeted enrollment of 11,000 women and a primary end point of maternal death or transfusion of packed red blood cells. Although this study is not specifically targeting PPH, the impact of prophylactic TXA on the subsequent incidence of PPH will add much needed information regarding this potential role for TXA use. Similarly, the TRAexaminc Acid For Preventing Postpartum Hemorrhage Following a Cesarean Delivery (TRAAP2) trial in France will take a similar approach with a targeted enrollment of 4524 women [32].

Liver transplantation surgery

Patients undergoing liver surgery or transplantation typically present with coagulation abnormalities, and hyperfibrinolysis is commonly seen, particularly during the anhepatic phase of transplantation [33]. The use of antifibrinolytics during orthotopic liver transplantation (OLT) was first introduced approximately 30 years ago and was shown to significantly decrease intraoperative blood loss and the use of platelets and cryoprecipitate [34]. Later, concerns were raised about the empiric use of antifibrinolytics and the risk of venous thromboembolism, including hepatic artery thrombosis and increased perioperative mortality [35]. Systemic fibrinolysis during OLT is frequently transient and not a major predictor of mortality, because it is associated with the late anhepatic and reperfusion stages when tPA is released from the vascular bed but is not yet cleared by the transplanted liver [36]. This finding has led to a more nuanced approach to the use of TXA in most transplant centers where viscoelastic hemostatic assay (VHA) monitoring (discussed in greater detail elsewhere in this article) is frequently used to guide the use of TXA when there is specific evidence of hyperfibrinolysis and bleeding.

An early meta-analysis done in 2007 looking at the safety and efficacy of antifibrinolytics in OLT found that both TXA and aprotinin reduced the need for transfusion without an associated increase in adverse outcomes, including thromboembolic events [37]. In their analysis, Molenaar and colleagues [37] looked at 23 studies with 1407 patients receiving either aprotinin, EACA, or TXA. A more recent Cochrane Systematic Review using a more rigorous interpretation of available data, however, found that only aprotinin accomplished these goals, with TXA only trending toward less blood loss and lower transfusion requirements [38].

Most recently, Badenoch and colleagues [39] reported on their single-center experience with TXA in a propensity-matched cohort study of 1799 consecutive liver transplant recipients. After propensity matching for confounders of transfusion and thrombotic risk, they identified 367 unique pairs for analysis. They found that patients receiving TXA (total dose of >10 mg/kg for 50% of the operative duration) received fewer allogenic blood transfusions (4 [1 (25th centile), 7 (75th centile)] for control group versus 3 [0, 6] for the TXA group) with no difference in thromboembolic events (22 [6.0%] for control group vs 36 [9.8%] for TXA group). These data represent the most recent assessment of TXA benefit during OLT and should reflect the changes in blood management during OLT that have occurred over the last 2 decades.

In summary, TXA continues to be used selectively for OLT surgery. The available evidence suggests there is likely a mild decrease in transfusion rates that is not associated with any other significant clinical outcomes. More important, despite concerns about an increased risk for thromboembolic events, all the larger studies and reviews have failed to identify this association as significant.

Orthopedic surgery

Minimizing blood loss and decreasing allogenic red blood cell transfusion in orthopedic surgery is also a topic of considerable interest. Blood transfusion during and after orthopedic surgery is associated with an increase in surgical site infections and increased costs [40], and therefore, measures to decrease overall blood loss and subsequent transfusion requirements are critical in the intraoperative and perioperative period. TXA has been extensively studied in this specialty population, specifically in hip [41,42] and knee arthroplasty [43,44], scoliosis operations [45,46], and after traumatic orthopedic injuries [40]. There are 3 primary questions with regard to TXA use in orthopedic surgery: (1) Does TXA administration improve outcomes, and if so, which outcomes?; (2) Via what route (ie, IV or topical) is TXA most beneficial?; and (3) Is there an optimal dose of TXA in orthopedic surgery?

The first question regarding efficacy of TXA in orthopedic surgery has been addressed in multiple prospective, randomized studies and subsequent meta-analyses. TXA has been shown to decrease the incidence and rate of red blood cell transfusion in primary hip [42] and knee arthroplasty [44]. Furthermore, there was no significant increased risk of thromboembolic complications noted with TXA use. In an adolescent scoliosis surgery population, Goobie and colleagues [46] reported in a prospective, randomized study that patients who received TXA had significantly lower volumes of blood loss and required significantly less intraoperative and postoperative blood transfusions. Finally, TXA has shown a significant association with decreased blood loss and transfusion requirements in operations for acute fractures. In a meta-analysis of patients who sustained traumatic orthopedic injuries that required operative intervention, Gausden and colleagues [40] reported that TXA was associated with a decreased risk of transfusion without a significant increase in thromboembolic complications.

Addressing the second question: Is there a route of TXA administration that is most beneficial for improved clinical outcomes? Previous investigations have evaluated topical (ie, intraarticular) TXA during hip [47] and knee arthroplasty [48,49]. Compared with placebo, TXA administration at the operative site significantly reduced the absolute risk of blood transfusion. Additionally, the TXA group had a significantly smaller decrease in postoperative hemoglobin as well as lower volumes of blood loss. Comparative studies evaluating topical TXA versus IV TXA have demonstrated noninferiority with regard to blood transfusion requirements, whereas combined topical and IV TXA compared with IV TXA was associated with improved outcomes [50]. Last, there is little evidence to guide optimal dosing of TXA in total joint arthroplasty. High-dose IV (>20 mg/kg or >1 g) or topical (>1.5 g) administration does not seem to be convincingly superior to low doses with respect to transfusion and blood loss after joint replacement. Overall, the American Academy of Orthopedic Surgeons provides a strong recommendation for the use of any administration of TXA for joint arthroplasty operations and states that it does not seem to increase the risk of thromboembolic or myocardial complications, although there is a recognized limited amount of adverse outcome data [51].

One of the interesting aspects of TXA use in orthopedic surgery is an association with postoperative wound infections. Although most studies were not powered to assess this interaction, there are several aspects of TXA usage that can influence surgical site infections. First, increased intraoperative transfusion requirements have been associated with an increased incidence of

injured patient during the prehospital and early management phases is a more recent development. Coagulation in trauma has received a considerable amount of attention and scientific investigation over the last 20 years. A pivotal investigation by Brohi and colleagues [70] identified that trauma induced coagulopathy (TIC) is present in nearly 25% of severely injured trauma patients and was associated with increased mortality. Much of this early work on TIC focused on traditional laboratory values, such as the prothrombin time, partial thromboplastin time, and the international normalized ratio [71]. However, these tests have several disadvantages, including the amount of time required to process the laboratory values and deliver the results, especially in clinical scenarios when early recognition of life-threatening hemorrhage and pathologic coagulation is paramount. In addition, traditional coagulation testing only measures isolated and separate coagulation pathways (ie, the intrinsic clotting pathway for partial thromboplastin time and the intrinsic pathway for prothrombin time/international normalized ratio) and does not directly assess for the presence of fibrinolysis. Recent evidence suggests that such conventional laboratory testing of coagulation does not provide the full picture of TIC and that a more sophisticated, cell-based model of coagulation testing would provide better overall clinical measures of coagulopathy after hemorrhage [72].

Severe trauma and associated hemorrhage contributes to a TIC that is mediated through various mechanisms, which results in coagulation factor depletion, platelet dysfunction, and fibrinolysis [73]. The underlying process by which dysregulated fibrinolysis proceeds is theorized to depend on the plasminogen pathway [74]. As previously noted, under normal physiologic conditions, plasminogen is converted to plasmin, which cleaves the fibrinogen meshwork upon which a hemostatic clot is formed. Pathologic fibrinolysis, as occurs in severe hemorrhagic shock and through activated protein C, leads to a release of tPA that increases subsequent levels of plasmin, which ultimately results in degradation of the formed clot [75]. This release of tPA is thought to be related to the severity of injury and depth of shock, such that hyperfibrinolysis is documented to occur in only a minority of severely injured trauma patients, but is associated with significantly increased transfusion requirements and mortality [76].

Fibrinolysis is most commonly measured in trauma patients with a VHA (discussed in greater detail elsewhere in this article), such as thromboelastography (TEG) or rotational thromboelastometry (ROTEM) [77]. Although fibrinolysis has been documented with ROTEM, it has been more commonly described with TEG (Fig. 3) [74,76,78,79]. Initial studies following traumatic injury defined significant and excessive fibrinolysis, or hyperfibrinolysis, as being present when the percentage of clot that lysed after 30 minutes (LY30) was 15% or greater. Although this was not an overall common phenotype, occurring in 11% of the highest-level trauma activations at a single trauma center, hyperfibrinolysis was associated with more frequent massive transfusion and significantly increased mortality [78] Further work by Cotton and colleagues

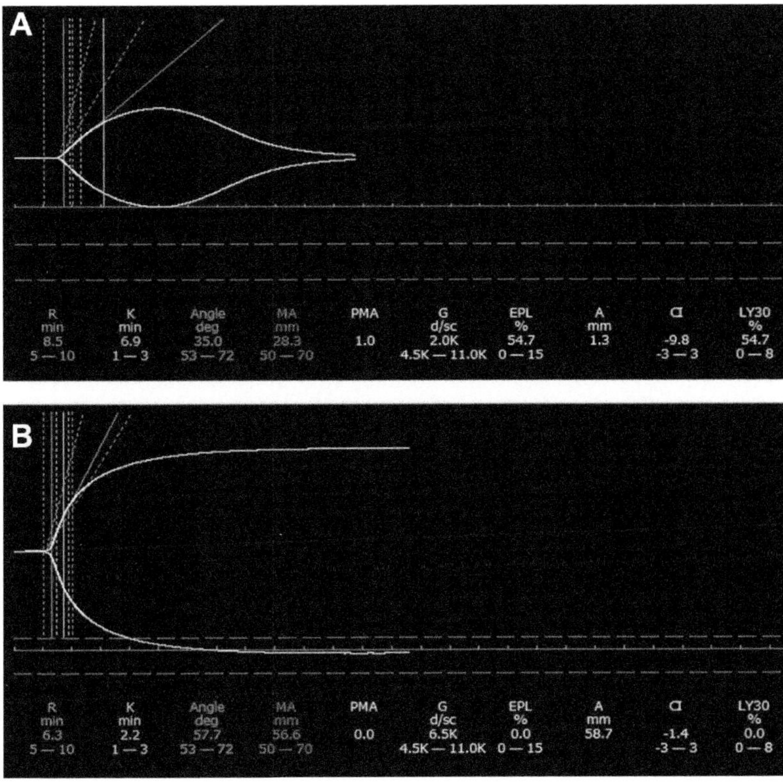

Fig. 3. Tracings obtained from TEG assessment during resuscitation in the setting of hemorrhagic shock and massive blood loss. (*A*) Hyperfibrinolysis evident during initial TEG with LY30 of 54.7%. (*B*) Reversal of hyperfibrinolysis approximately 30 minutes following administration of TXA (1 g over 10 minutes) with concomitant use of cryoprecipitate, fresh frozen plasma, packed red blood cells during massive resuscitation protocol.

[76] used an LY30 of greater than 7.5% with rapid TEG to define hyperfibrinolysis and observed an incidence of 2% in a population of 1996 trauma patients. This definition of hyperfibrinolysis was associated with worse injury severity, greater depth of shock, increased transfusion requirements, and significantly worse mortality. Furthermore, the authors noted that greater prehospital crystalloid administration was a significant risk factor for hyperfibrinolysis, providing further questions into the underlying etiology of this coagulopathic phenomenon. More recent studies have demonstrated that an even lower threshold of hyperfibrinolysis is clinically relevant. Chapman and colleagues [80] described an LY30 of greater than 3% as accurately identifying patients with hyperfibrinolysis, and, similar to prior investigations, this finding was associated with significantly increased transfusion requirements and mortality. These findings were corroborated by other investigators using data from the Pragmatic, Randomized, Optimal Platelet and Plasma ratio (PROPPr) trial

[81]. The authors described fibrinolysis in 3 categories (discussed in greater detail elsewhere in this article) and noted that hyperfibrinolysis, defined as an LY30 of greater than 3%, was associated with worse injury severity, depth of shock, coagulopathy, increased blood product transfusion requirements, and worse 24-hour and 30-day mortality. To date, the entirety of available data clearly shows that hyperfibrinolysis after traumatic injury is a clinically important entity that is associated with worse outcomes.

Tranexamic acid and traumatic injury

This association of hyperfibrinolysis and worse outcomes along with a potential role for the early use of antifibrinolytics in the setting of TIC led to the pivotal CRASH-2 trial [6]. This often-quoted study included adult trauma patients with, or at risk of, significant bleeding, randomly assigned within 8 hours of injury to either TXA (loading dose of 1 g IV over 10 minutes then an infusion of 1 g over 8 hours) or placebo groups. The primary outcome was 28-day in-hospital mortality with a total enrollment of 10,060 patients in the TXA group and 10,067 in the placebo group. All-cause mortality was significantly decreased with TXA (1463 [14.5%] vs 1613 [16.0%] in the control group; RR, 0.85; 95% CI, 0.85–0.97; $P = .0035$) as was the risk of death owing to bleeding (489 [4.9%] vs 574 [5.7%] in the placebo group; RR, 0.85; 95% CI, 0.76–0.96; $P = .007$). A secondary analysis of the patients who died from bleeding found that the benefit from TXA was greatest when it was given early ($\leq$1 hour) after injury with a paradoxic increase in death when given more than 3 hours after injury [82]. Early criticisms of the CRASH-2 trial noted that fewer than 2% of the patients were treated in countries that routinely provide rapid access to blood products, damage control surgery, angiography, and advanced critical care. Subsequent work suggests that the early use of TXA in a mature trauma system may not improve outcomes in most patients [83–86]. Taken together, the CRASH-2 trial and these more recent studies continue to engender controversy regarding the role of TXA in acute trauma [87–91].

Other major studies supporting a role for TXA in the early resuscitation come from recent combat casualty management. The Military Application of Tranexamic Acid in Trauma Emergency Resuscitation (MATTERs) and MATTERs II trials have offered further insight into the role of TXA in patients requiring massive transfusion in a military setting [92,93]. The former study retrospectively evaluated 896 patients receiving a blood transfusion at a single surgical military hospital in southern Afghanistan from January 1, 2009, to December 31, 2010. The authors reported that, despite being more severely injured, patients who received TXA (1 g bolus administered based on the requirement of emergency blood product transfusion or evidence of hyperfibrinolysis on viscoelastic testing) experienced an improved 48-hour and in-hospital mortality rate [93]. The improved clinical outcomes were also present in those patients requiring a massive transfusion, defined as 10 or more units red blood cells in 24 hours. Additionally, there was no association between TXA use and thromboembolic complications. Interestingly, a more recent review of the US military experience with TXA identified an association between TXA use and venous thromboembolism as an independent risk factor (odds ratio, 2.58; 95% CI, 1.20–5.56; $P = .02$). This finding is not consistent with the CRASH-2 or MATTERs trials, but may reflect the unique military patient population, which has a higher incidence of deep vein thrombosis and frequently requires extended medical evacuation with longer periods of immobility [94].

Further work by the same authors in the MATTERs II trial evaluated the concomitant administration of cryoprecipitate with TXA in a similar military population of wounded patients [92]. Despite population heterogeneity, with patients who received cryoprecipitate and TXA being more severely injured, these patients demonstrated the lowest mortality rate of the study cohort. These results support a more selective role for TXA use in severe trauma and highlight the likely importance of other factors in addressing TIC. The role of specific factors such as cryoprecipitate and fibrinogen continue to be examined in ongoing work. Moore and colleagues [95] found that early plasma administration attenuated the effects of hyperfibrinolysis in an animal model of hemorrhagic shock. This finding is critical because fibrinogen is the first coagulation factor to be depleted and reach critically low levels after severe hemorrhage [96]. Therefore, replacement of fibrinogen, with cryoprecipitate or fibrinogen concentrates (as is commonly performed in European trauma systems), in combination with TXA may serve to treat severe fibrinogen deficiency as well as promote clot stabilization with inhibition of plasminogen activity. However, further scientific work examining the precise role of TXA in trauma is necessary because resuscitation from hemorrhagic shock moves toward a goal-directed approach of correcting the specific derangements in coagulation [97].

Beyond the impact of treating fibrinolysis, the benefit of TXA use in the trauma patient receiving care in a dedicated mature trauma system may have other roles. The mechanism of action related to early administration and previously described survival benefit continues to be examined. Recent studies suggest an alternate or contributing mechanism related to preservation of the endothelial glycocalyx in shock and other acute injury states [98]. In an animal model, Kozar and colleagues [99] found that hemorrhagic shock injures the endothelial glycocalyx, which can be restored by plasma, but not lactated Ringers solution, resuscitation. Other data suggest that glycocalyx shedding contributes to vascular permeability in severely injured trauma patients [100]. Diebel and colleagues [101] have demonstrated in vitro that TXA may exert a protective influence on the glycocalyx in a shock model using human umbilical vein. This model suggests that the role for TXA in the trauma patient may be multifactorial and not exclusive to its antifibrinolytic properties. It also supports the previously reported observation that earlier administration achieves greater effect. Not all work, however, has supported these findings [102]. Despite all of the existing evidence, TXA use in trauma is variable throughout United States [103].

Viscoelastic assessment of fibrinolysis in trauma

Use of a VHA represents an alternative means of measuring a cell-based model of coagulation and hold several advantages over traditional coagulation tests for the traumatically injured patient [72,97]. TEG and ROTEM are VHAs that have been described to measure the various components of TIC and specific deficiencies in hemostatic coagulation. TEG is the most commonly described VHA in trauma centers in the United States, whereas ROTEM is frequently used throughout trauma centers in Europe. Although comparison studies of these 2 VHAs demonstrate that their results are not interchangeable [104], both tests provide potentially useful information that is associated with clinical outcomes in patients with hemorrhage [105]. Both viscoelastic tests use a sample of citrated whole blood placed in a cuvette; the whole blood sample is then activated with either calcium chloride or kaolin, in the example of ROTEM and TEG, respectively. Following sample agitation and clot initiation the time and strength of clot formation is measured by tension generated on a wire that is immersed in the sample of whole blood. The natural physiologic regulation of hemostatic clot formation is eventual clot lysis and dissolution. In the case of TEG, clot lysis is measured as the LY30 after the maximum clot amplitude is achieved [106].

As noted, clot dissolution is a physiologic and regulated response of coagulation so that hemostasis is appropriately achieved, but that clot is not excessively and inappropriately produced, resulting in widespread and unregulated thrombosis. Traditional measures of clot lysis, such as fibrin split products and the D-dimer test, have previously been used to diagnose more frequently discussed fibrinolytic pathology, such as disseminated intravascular coagulation. However, like other conventional tests of coagulation, there is a significant disadvantage of these laboratory values in the acutely hemorrhaging patient because of the prolonged delay in obtaining these results [107].

When the decision is made to use TXA, the question remains, "Is there a therapeutic target to correct hyperfibrinolysis?" Although data from the CRASH-2 [6] and MATTERs [93] studies address TXA administration to improve mortality as a result of hemorrhage after trauma, neither of these investigations provided viscoelastic data to demonstrate that hyperfibrinolysis was present in these patients and to what extent TXA may have impacted the outcome in patients with pathologic clot lysis. Recent evidence also demonstrates that there are numerous proteomic mechanisms at play in patients with hyperfibrinolysis. Although it was previously mentioned that the activated protein C pathway is integral to TIC and the subsequent activation of tPA, Banerjee and colleagues [108] noted that a variety of coagulation proteins are decreased in patients with hyperfibrinolysis, most notably antiprotease proteins in addition to proteins that reflect activation of the complement system. In aggregate, hyperfibrinolysis is a highly integrated phenomenon with multiple underlying components that respond to severe injury and shock to produce the release of tPA and promote clot instability.

Because TXA is more critically explored in severely injured trauma patients, our understanding of the fibrinolytic process is expanding. There exists the question of whether TXA is warranted and beneficial in every trauma patient in whom there is suspicion of hemorrhage. Recent evidence would suggest that TXA use may be harmful in certain patients, based on TEG data obtained upon admission to the trauma centers [83,90]. Physiologic fibrinolysis has now been frequently used to identify the protective effect of certain, but limited, fibrinolysis activity to maintain vascular patency. On one end of the fibrinolysis spectrum is hyperfibrinolysis, identified as an LY30 of greater than 3%, whereas on the other and opposite end is fibrinolysis shutdown, defined as an LY30 of less than 0.8%. This terminology, consisting of fibrinolysis shutdown, physiologic fibrinolysis, and hyperfibrinolysis, has been reported in the trauma literature [79,81]. Although hyperfibrinolysis is associated with significantly increased mortality, there is also retrospective evidence to suggest that patients in fibrinolysis shutdown also experience an increased mortality burden that is attributed to multiple organ failure [109]. It is unclear based on the level of evidence if this increased mortality is the direct result of TXA administration, resulting in fibrinolysis shutdown or the pathophysiologic response to tissue injury. Nonetheless, there is retrospective evidence of an association of increased mortality in patients with physiologic fibrinolysis who receive TXA [83]. Considering the present evidence in the trauma literature, there is increasing support for selective use of TXA in trauma patients based on viscoelastic data gathered on arrival to the trauma center [110].

Ongoing research on tranexamic acid and trauma

Currently, several ongoing, prospective trials may shed some light on the usefulness of TXA for severely injured patients at risk of TIC based on their fibrinolytic phenotype. The Pre-hospital Anti-Fibrinolytics for Traumatic Coagulopathy & Haemorrhage (PATCH-Trauma Study) is currently underway in Australia and New Zealand as a multicenter, randomized, double-blind, placebo-controlled trial of prehospital treatment with TXA [111]. This study includes a more extensive assessment of fibrinolysis than was done with CRASH-2 and should provide critical insights into the interplay between fibrinolytic states and TXA administration for severe trauma. Similarly, in the United States, the Study of Tranexamic Acid during Aeromedical Prehospital Transport (STAAMP) trial is underway to evaluate the effect of prehospital TXA administered during air medical transport and shortly after hospital admission in a randomized, controlled study [112]. The inclusion of a VHA in both studies will address some of the existing knowledge gaps regarding TXA use and fibrinolytic states in the prehospital setting. A third multicenter, prehospital study has completed enrollment evaluating the use of TXA for patients with suspected traumatic brain injury (moderate to severe) receiving TXA with a 1-g bolus followed by an additional 1 g over 8 hours compared with a 2-g bolus or placebo [113]. This study is more focused on neurologic outcomes, but will provide some data regarding the coagulopathic state of enrolled patients.

One other ongoing trial may provide additional data to guide the use of TXA in trauma patients. The Tranexamic Acid Mechanisms and Pharmacokinetics in Traumatic Injury (TAMPITI) Trial being conducted at a single center trial in the United States will assess higher dose TXA administration (a 2- or 4-g IV bolus) [114]. The primary end points in this trial are safety and efficacy with a focus on anti-inflammatory markers rather than coagulation status that may not address the question of TXA usage in the setting of shutdown.

SUMMARY

Antifibrinolytic therapy is increasingly being used in the perioperative setting as part of a blood conservation strategy or for management of bleeding in trauma and PPH. Although TXA has been used in OLT and cardiac surgery patients for a number of years, it has been suggested that it should be considered for any surgery where the expected blood loss is greater than 500 mL [115]. This agent has certainly been adopted widely for major orthopedic and spine surgery and is supported by recent studies with no evidence of increased thromboembolic events. Current areas of controversy seem to be centered around the role of TXA in trauma and PPH despite massive trials showing benefit. These areas of controversy primarily focus on the likely risk-benefit when TXA is used in a mature medical system with early access to surgical options, readily available blood product support, and advanced care options as compared with low- or medium-resource environments. In the area of early trauma management, research on the interaction of antifibrinolytic therapy and fibrinolytic shutdown has also brought out other questions regarding timing and appropriateness of TXA for subsets of bleeding trauma patients. Ongoing research in these areas will provide a better understanding of the benefits of early antifibrinolytic use for these specific patient populations in the next several years.

References

[1] Ro JS, Knutrud O, Stormorken H. Antifibrinolytic treatment with tranexamic acid (AMCA) in pediatric urinary tract surgery. J Pediatr Surg 1970;5(3):315–20.

[2] Vermylen J, Verhaegen-Declercq ML, Verstraete M, et al. A double blind study of the effect of tranexamic acid in essential menorrhagia. Thromb Diath Haemorrh 1968;20(3): 583–7.

[3] Okamoto S, Sato S, Takada Y, et al. An active stereo-isomer (trans-form) of Amcha and its antifibrinolytic (antiplasminic) action in vitro and in vivo. Keio J Med 1964;13:177–85.

[4] Melander B, Gliniecki G, Granstrand B, et al. Biochemistry and toxicology of amikapron; the antifibrinolytically active isomer of AMCHA. (A comparative study with epsilon-aminocaproic acid). Acta Pharmacol Toxicol (Copenh) 1965;22(4):340–52.

[5] World Health Organization. WHO model list of essential medicines, 20th edition (March 2017, amended August 2017). Geneva (Switzerland): World Health Organization; 2017.

[6] CRASH-2 Trial Collaborators. Effects of tranexamic acid on death, vascular occlusive events, and blood transfusion in trauma patients with significant haemorrhage (CRASH-2): a randomised, placebo-controlled trial. Lancet 2010;376(9734):23–32.

[7] Woman Trial Collaborators. Effect of early tranexamic acid administration on mortality, hysterectomy, and other morbidities in women with post-partum haemorrhage (WOMAN): an international, randomised, double-blind, placebo-controlled trial. Lancet 2017;389(10084):2105–16.
[8] Vogel JP, Oladapo OT, Dowswell T, et al. Updated WHO recommendation on intravenous tranexamic acid for the treatment of post-partum haemorrhage. Lancet Glob Health 2018;6(1):e18–9.
[9] Schneeweiss S, Seeger JD, Landon J, et al. Aprotinin during coronary-artery bypass grafting and risk of death. N Engl J Med 2008;358(8):771–83.
[10] Shaw AD, Stafford-Smith M, White WD, et al. The effect of aprotinin on outcome after coronary-artery bypass grafting. N Engl J Med 2008;358(8):784–93.
[11] Trasylol (aprotinin)-important new safety information-for the public. 2011. Available at: http://healthycanadians.gc.ca/recall-alert-rappel-avis/hc-sc/2011/14107a-eng.php. Accessed June 23, 2019.
[12] European Medicines Agency. Assessment report: antifibrinolytics containing aprotinin, aminocaproic acid and tranexamic acid. 2013. Available at: https://www.ema.europa.eu/en/documents/referral/assessment-report-antifibrinolytic-medicines-aprotinin_en.pdf. Accessed June 23, 2019.
[13] Benedetto U, Altman DG, Gerry S, et al. Safety of perioperative aprotinin administration during isolated coronary artery bypass graft surgery: insights from the ART (Arterial Revascularization Trial). J Am Heart Assoc 2018;7(5):e007570.
[14] Wu G, Mazzitelli BA, Quek AJ, et al. Tranexamic acid is an active site inhibitor of urokinase plasminogen activator. Blood Adv 2019;3(5):729–33.
[15] Medcalf RL. The traumatic side of fibrinolysis. Blood 2015;125(16):2457–8.
[16] Reed R, Woolley T. Uses of tranexamic acid. Cont Educ Anaesth Crit Care Pain 2015;15(1):32–7.
[17] Gupta S, Bhiwal AK, Karuna S. Tranexamic acid: beware of anaesthetic misadventures. J Obstet Anaesth Crit Care 2018;8(1):1–6.
[18] Eriksson O, Kjellman H, Schannong M. The biological availability of Cyklokapron tablets compared with Cyklokapron solution administered orally. Stockholm (Sweden): Kabi AB; 1971.
[19] Picetti R, Shakur-Still H, Medcalf RL, et al. What concentration of tranexamic acid is needed to inhibit fibrinolysis? A systematic review of pharmacodynamics studies. Blood Coagul Fibrinolysis 2019;30(1):1–10.
[20] Kullander S, Nilsson IM. Human placental transfer of an antifibrinolytic agent (AMCA). Acta Obstet Gynecol Scand 1970;49(3):241–2.
[21] Ahlberg A, Eriksson O, Kjellman H. Diffusion of tranexamic acid to the joint. Acta Orthop Scand 1976;47(5):486–8.
[22] Nilsson IM. Clinical pharmacology of aminocaproic and tranexamic acids. J Clin Pathol Suppl (R Coll Pathol) 1980;14:41–7.
[23] Jerath A, Yang QJ, Pang KS, et al. Tranexamic acid dosing for cardiac surgical patients with chronic renal dysfunction: a new dosing regimen. Anesth Analg 2018;127(6):1323–32.
[24] Montroy J, Hutton B, Moodley P, et al. The efficacy and safety of topical tranexamic acid: a systematic review and meta-analysis. Trans Med Rev 2018;32(3):165–78.
[25] Kassebaum NJ, Bertozzi-Villa A, Coggeshall MS, et al. Global, regional, and national levels and causes of maternal mortality during 1990-2013: a systematic analysis for the Global Burden of Disease Study 2013. Lancet 2014;384(9947):980–1004.
[26] Allard S, Green L, Hunt BJ. How we manage the haematological aspects of major obstetric haemorrhage. Br J Haematol 2014;164(2):177–88.
[27] Pacheco LD, Saade GR, Costantine MM, et al. An update on the use of massive transfusion protocols in obstetrics. Am J Obstet Gynecol 2016;214(3):340–4.

[28] Heesen M, Bohmer J, Klohr S, et al. Prophylactic tranexamic acid in parturients at low risk for post-partum haemorrhage: systematic review and meta-analysis. Acta Anaesthesiol Scand 2014;58(9):1075–85.
[29] Ducloy-Bouthors AS, Jude B, Duhamel A, et al. High-dose tranexamic acid reduces blood loss in postpartum haemorrhage. Crit Care 2011;15(2):R117.
[30] Committee on Practice Bulletins-Obstetrics. Practice bulletin no. 183: postpartum hemorrhage. Obstet Gynecol 2017;130(4):e168–86.
[31] The George Washington University Biostatistics Center. Tranexamic acid for the prevention of obstetrical hemorrhage after cesarean section (TXA). 2019. Available at: https://clinicaltrials.gov/ct2/show/NCT03364491. Accessed June 26, 2019.
[32] TRAnexamic acid for preventing postpartum hemorrhage following a cesarean delivery (TRAAP2). 2019. Available at: https://clinicaltrials.gov/ct2/show/NCT03431805?recrs=a&cond=obstetrical+hemorrhage. Accessed June 25, 2019.
[33] Roullet S, Pillot J, Freyburger G, et al. Rotation thromboelastometry detects thrombocytopenia and hypofibrinogenaemia during orthotopic liver transplantation. Br J Anaesth 2010;104(4):422–8.
[34] Boylan JF, Klinck JR, Sandler AN, et al. Tranexamic acid reduces blood loss, transfusion requirements, and coagulation factor use in primary orthotopic liver transplantation. Anesthesiology 1996;85(5):1043–8 [discussion: 1030A–1A].
[35] Xia VW, Steadman RH. Antifibrinolytics in orthotopic liver transplantation: current status and controversies. Liver Transpl 2005;11(1):10–8.
[36] Kang Y, Audu P. Coagulation and liver transplantation. Int Anesthesiol Clin 2006;44(4): 17–36.
[37] Molenaar IQ, Warnaar N, Groen H, et al. Efficacy and safety of antifibrinolytic drugs in liver transplantation: a systematic review and meta-analysis. Am J Transplant 2007;7(1):185–94.
[38] Gurusamy KS, Pissanou T, Pikhart H, et al. Methods to decrease blood loss and transfusion requirements for liver transplantation. Cochrane Database Syst Rev 2011;(12):CD009052.
[39] Badenoch A, Sharma A, Gower S, et al. The effectiveness and safety of tranexamic acid in orthotopic liver transplantation clinical practice: a propensity score matched cohort study. Transplantation 2017;101(7):1658–65.
[40] Gausden EB, Qudsi R, Boone MD, et al. Tranexamic acid in orthopaedic trauma surgery: a meta-analysis. J Orthop Trauma 2017;31(10):513–9.
[41] Lee C, Freeman R, Edmondson M, et al. The efficacy of tranexamic acid in hip hemiarthroplasty surgery: an observational cohort study. Injury 2015;46(10):1978–82.
[42] Zufferey PJ, Miquet M, Quenet S, et al. Tranexamic acid in hip fracture surgery: a randomized controlled trial. Br J Anaesth 2010;104(1):23–30.
[43] Cid J, Lozano M. Tranexamic acid reduces allogeneic red cell transfusions in patients undergoing total knee arthroplasty: results of a meta-analysis of randomized controlled trials. Transfusion 2005;45(8):1302–7.
[44] Yang ZG, Chen WP, Wu LD. Effectiveness and safety of tranexamic acid in reducing blood loss in total knee arthroplasty: a meta-analysis. J Bone Joint Surg Am 2012;94(13): 1153–9.
[45] Cheriyan T, Maier SP 2nd, Bianco K, et al. Efficacy of tranexamic acid on surgical bleeding in spine surgery: a meta-analysis. Spine J 2015;15(4):752–61.
[46] Goobie SM, Zurakowski D, Glotzbecker MP, et al. Tranexamic acid is efficacious at decreasing the rate of blood loss in adolescent scoliosis surgery: a randomized placebo-controlled trial. J Bone Joint Surg Am 2018;100(23):2024–32.
[47] Alshryda S, Mason J, Sarda P, et al. Topical (intra-articular) tranexamic acid reduces blood loss and transfusion rates following total hip replacement: a randomized controlled trial (TRANX-H). J Bone Joint Surg Am 2013;95(21):1969–74.

[48] Alshryda S, Mason J, Vaghela M, et al. Topical (intra-articular) tranexamic acid reduces blood loss and transfusion rates following total knee replacement: a randomized controlled trial (TRANX-K). J Bone Joint Surg Am 2013;95(21):1961–8.
[49] Abdel MP, Chalmers BP, Taunton MJ, et al. Intravenous versus topical tranexamic acid in total knee arthroplasty: both effective in a randomized clinical trial of 640 patients. J Bone Joint Surg Am 2018;100(12):1023–9.
[50] Gomez-Barrena E, Ortega-Andreu M, Padilla-Eguiluz NG, et al. Topical intra-articular compared with intravenous tranexamic acid to reduce blood loss in primary total knee replacement: a double-blind, randomized, controlled, noninferiority clinical trial. J Bone Joint Surg Am 2014;96(23):1937–44.
[51] Fillingham YA, Ramkumar DB, Jevsevar DS, et al. Tranexamic acid in total joint arthroplasty: the endorsed clinical practice guides of the American Association of Hip and Knee Surgeons, American Society of Regional Anesthesia and Pain Medicine, American Academy of Orthopaedic Surgeons, Hip Society, and Knee Society. Reg Anesth Pain Med 2019;44(1):7–11.
[52] Bernard AC, Davenport DL, Chang PK, et al. Intraoperative transfusion of 1 U to 2 U packed red blood cells is associated with increased 30-day mortality, surgical-site infection, pneumonia, and sepsis in general surgery patients. J Am Coll Surg 2009;208(5): 931–7, 937.e931-932; [discussion: 938–9].
[53] Rhee C, Lethbridge L, Richardson G, et al. Risk factors for infection, revision, death, blood transfusion and longer hospital stay 3 months and 1 year after primary total hip or knee arthroplasty. Can J Surg 2018;61(3):165–76.
[54] Klasan A, Dworschak P, Heyse TJ, et al. Transfusions increase complications and infections after hip and knee arthroplasty: an analysis of 2760 cases. Technol Health Care 2018;26(5):825–32.
[55] Hart A, Khalil JA, Carli A, et al. Blood transfusion in primary total hip and knee arthroplasty. Incidence, risk factors, and thirty-day complication rates. J Bone Joint Surg Am 2014;96(23):1945–51.
[56] Pauzenberger L, Domej MA, Heuberer PR, et al. The effect of intravenous tranexamic acid on blood loss and early post-operative pain in total shoulder arthroplasty. Bone Joint J 2017;99-B(8):1073–9.
[57] Cordero-Ampuero J, de Dios M. What are the risk factors for infection in hemiarthroplasties and total hip arthroplasties? Clin Orthop Relat Res 2010;468(12):3268–77.
[58] Levy JH, Koster A, Quinones QJ, et al. Antifibrinolytic therapy and perioperative considerations. Anesthesiology 2018;128(3):657–70.
[59] Draxler DF, Yep K, Hanafi G, et al. Tranexamic acid modulates the immune response and reduces postsurgical infection rates. Blood Adv 2019;3(10):1598–609.
[60] Koster A, Faraoni D, Levy JH. Antifibrinolytic therapy for cardiac surgery: an update. Anesthesiology 2015;123(1):214–21.
[61] Horrow JC, Van Riper DF, Strong MD, et al. The dose-response relationship of tranexamic acid. Anesthesiology 1995;82(2):383–92.
[62] Fiechtner BK, Nuttall GA, Johnson ME, et al. Plasma tranexamic acid concentrations during cardiopulmonary bypass. Anesth Analg 2001;92(5):1131–6.
[63] Nuttall GA, Gutierrez MC, Dewey JD, et al. A preliminary study of a new tranexamic acid dosing schedule for cardiac surgery. J Cardiothorac Vasc Anesth 2008;22(2):230–5.
[64] Dowd NP, Karski JM, Cheng DC, et al. Pharmacokinetics of tranexamic acid during cardiopulmonary bypass. Anesthesiology 2002;97(2):390–9.
[65] Sigaut S, Tremey B, Ouattara A, et al. Comparison of two doses of tranexamic acid in adults undergoing cardiac surgery with cardiopulmonary bypass. Anesthesiology 2014;120(3):590–600.
[66] Myles PS, Smith JA, Forbes A, et al. Tranexamic acid in patients undergoing coronary-artery surgery. N Engl J Med 2017;376(2):136–48.

are compelling words about the joys and advantages of working as an anesthesiologist in several different practice situations. All are meaningful work. All provide an individual the opportunity to practice medicine at the cutting edge of anesthesiology, pain management, or critical care. All offer a pathway to a rewarding career. The differences lie in the daily details, but the essential work is similar.

Academic anesthesiology is unique. The academic anesthesiologist has all the same clinical opportunities as his or her colleagues in private practice, and maybe more. Academic medical centers frequently care for complex patients at the extremes of physiology undergoing high-risk, or sometimes even experimental, surgery. In essence, the clinical duties are similar. Academic anesthesiologists are assigned to care for a patient, review the patient's records, greet the patient, establish rapport, and plan an anesthetic. The individual is cared for through all phases of the perioperative journey. Academic anesthesiologists prescribe medications, perform technical procedures, attend at the bedside in the OR, guide enhanced recovery care pathways, and participate in extended care when, and where, necessary. Through their hands, academic anesthesiologists are the sentinel of safety for the patient. There is no distance between the role the academic anesthesiologist plays in clinical patient care and that of colleagues in private practice; in fact, academic anesthesiologists are more likely to engage in collateral activities such as critical care. What makes academic anesthesiology unique is the extension of the work to include the educational and research mission of their specialty.

The academic anesthesiologist contributes to a good much greater than himself or herself. The scholarly pursuits of creating new knowledge (eg, research) and transmission of this knowledge to others (eg, education) extend the work of the academic anesthesiologist a step beyond that of clinical care alone. This participation in scholarship is the fuel that inspires the academic anesthesiologist to work long hours, even after the surgical theater is empty. The participation in scholarship provides an immortal contribution that is sometimes visible to all, as in a publication, while at other times, invisible even to the academic physician. Who among us, though, does not recall our mentors, our teachers, and those from whom we learned the techniques and tricks that have saved another's life? In those moments, sometimes decades after the fact, the student will recall the teacher. Knowing that our actions today will affect a generation of physicians tomorrow is a rich reward for the academic anesthesiologist, a reward that provides deep meaning to the work.

The educational mission

Most academic anesthesiologists are clinician-educators. The educational construct relies on an apprentice-style learning in which the novice physician meets certain competency milestones while they mature across the continuum of residency toward proficiency. The clinician-educator plays a vital role in this educational continuum. On day 1, the experience of the learner is minimal and the guidance and tutelage from the clinician-educator must be near total. As training progresses, the clinician-educator allows for increasing autonomy, while always maintaining ultimate responsibility. To see a novice physician progress toward competence is one of the great rewards of this work.

This apprentice style learning in a residency program is only 1 component of the educational mission. An academic anesthesiologist is usually expected to deliver lectures, hold seminars, host workshops, and provide other didactic works that complement intraoperative teaching. These products of scholarship may be for an audience of a few (eg, small group discussions) or thousands (eg, meeting presentations). Often, the academic anesthesiologist will produce durable works of scholarship (eg, publications) in this educational domain to include case reports, manuscript reviews, book chapters, books, and original research.

There are 142 residency training programs in the United States, with an estimated 7500 residents in training and an estimated 7000 academic anesthesiologists in this workforce. Of the approximately 46,000 practicing anesthesiologists in the country, about 1 in 7 is engaged in academia [9].

The research mission

Most academic anesthesiologists are not involved in true research. However, many, if not all, support the research mission through their support of the infrastructure that is required for research. This support includes an indirect financial contribution by each faculty physician (eg, via clinical revenue generation) to support unfunded, nascent research in the department. Cleary, an argument for moving to private practice is that, "I can do the same work and make more money!" Yes, in many instances the private practitioner makes more money in terms of cash compensation (although this gap is narrowing), but it is not for the same work. The work is fundamentally different, and the motivations and satisfactions are different. In addition, academic anesthesiologists are typically employed by a medical school, which can often provide noncash compensation benefits (eg, insurance packages, retirement options, or child tuition expenses) at or above those offered by private practice groups.

In 2018, anesthesiology as a specialty received $157.4 million in National Institutes of Health research awards as well as additional external funding from the Department of Defense and other federal agencies. Additional nongovernmental research support is also provided to anesthesiology departments from other agencies and corporations, such as the Anesthesia Patient Safety Foundation, the Foundation for Anesthesia Education and Research, and numerous technological and pharmaceutical companies. Who does the research work, and where does it occur?

The creation of new knowledge is one of the most important and satisfying roles of the academic anesthesiologist. The gains in safety for our patients and the advances in medications we administer today that render a patient unconscious and/or insensate arose through the work of physician researchers and their PhD colleagues. The original observations at the bedside, inspiring the work at the bench, and then the subsequent validation through participation in clinical trials are the product of scientific effort. We should never surrender this unique and identifying element of being a physician anesthesiologist. Those in academics are the contributing agents of this great purpose. The participation in this work gives life meaning.

The future of academic anesthesiology

The future of academic anesthesiology is bright (Table 1). Although care at the bedside evolves to include a greater degree of participation by nonphysician clinicians, the physician's roles as the formative educator and innovative researcher remain essential. The challenge for academic programs is to learn to economically compete in a changing landscape of professional reimbursement while maintaining lines of funding for education and research. Although at times this funding problem seems insurmountable, it is not. The postulate that our society can abandon the fundamental missions of education and

Table 1
Benefits and risks of practice in an academic department

Pros	Cons
High-quality noncash compensation and benefits (eg, retirement packages, insurance plans, malpractice coverage, dependent tuition assistance)	Potentially lower cash compensation
Opportunity to conduct research	Production pressure to produce nonclinical products (eg, publications, presentations)
Opportunity to train future anesthesiologists	Production pressure to create and deliver educational content to learners
Ability to receive promotions based on clinical and scholarly achievements	Clinical revenue generated by the department "taxed" by the medical school to maintain infrastructure
Often given protected nonclinical time to pursue scholarly activity	At times multiple layers of leadership in the institution may lead to slow progress/change
Typical anesthesia care team clinical care ratios are lower	Areas of greatest anesthesia practice expansion are in non-OR locations, which may be less professionally satisfying
Greater ability to focus on a clinical concentration (eg, pediatric, cardiothoracic, or regional anesthesia)	
Ability to create robust patient safety and quality improvement program infrastructure	
Robust infrastructure for regulatory reporting, usually through the hospital system	
The work contributes to the greater good, not just the bottom line financially	
Most practices have high-quality electronic medical records for anesthesia care record (eg, EPIC, Cerner)	
Well-established HR departments with clear guidelines and procedures for protecting employees	

research is a false one. Clearly, a society may choose to not fund these missions, but such an errant decision is soon unmasked and amended. The appetite we have as a species to improve our current condition will not, in the long run, allow the abandonment of the education and research mission.

As to the individual, there will always be the draw of an academic career. In academic practice, one can pursue a higher ideal. One attains the satisfaction of clinical care, as do our colleagues in private practice, but we also fully participate in the ideals of a higher scholarly pursuit. The creation of knowledge and the dissemination of that knowledge to the next generation are magical. If, as Frankl postulates, life's meaning arises through love, courage, and good work, then choosing the life of an academic anesthesiologist will always be a valuable option. This is good work.

SMALL- TO MEDIUM-SIZED GROUP PARTNERSHIP

Introduction

Small- to medium-sized private practice anesthesiology groups are enduring models for patient care. The dream of "hanging a shingle" and caring for patients is an iconic concept for many physicians. This practice model encompasses the spectrum of anesthesiology care, including traditional operating suite, intensive care unit, obstetrics, and pain management. Sustainable smaller practices are continually evolving and maturing organizationally to meet the needs of modern practice and embrace newer care models.

Benefits

Small- to medium-sized anesthesiology practices deliver a significant proportion of anesthetic care in the United States; the authors estimate that roughly 15% of all cases are done in academic centers, 20% by clinicians in large groups and the remainder by small- to medium-sized private practice groups (defined as <200 anesthesiologists; [Richard P. Dutton, MD MBA, personal communication, 2019], US Anesthesia Partners). The principal focus of private practice anesthesiology groups is providing high-quality patient care in a local area. The patient-physician relationship is strong, and these physicians gain satisfaction from a familiar clinical "family." The private practitioner's work time is without professional distractions, such as the need to perform research or publish. These physicians are dedicated to their practice, have a sense of ownership, and intuitively understand the need to promote their practice's brand.

Financial incentives are a salient factor enticing anesthesiologists into smaller private practices. Although incomes vary, private practitioners are generally well compensated for their services. Beyond the monetary benefits, private practitioners have flexibility over their daily schedule, call schedule, case mix, vacation, and meeting time. Depending on the setting, monetary and nonmonetary benefits can exceed those in academic- or large-practice settings. Smaller practices can also realize economic efficiencies and cost containment not available to larger groups. For example, the ability to outsource operational services, such as payroll, can result in reduction of fixed overhead expense.

Small- to medium-sized private practices are focused on the practice and its individual members. The model is highly flexible and able to meet both the interests of members and the needs of patients. The practice can influence multiple aspects, including sites of service, collaborating surgeons, and specialty areas of practice. In addition, the organization can select a practice model best suited to the members. Options include solo practice, a care team model, or any combination. Practices can choose to affiliate with academic institutions and participate in teaching anesthesiology to medical students, residents, or other types of trainees. Many practices promote specialty care across the spectrum of anesthesia care specialties, including traditional operating suite, intensive care, cardiac, pediatric, obstetric, and pain.

In addition to the practice's influence, individual anesthesiologists also have substantial control over their practice environment. This influence begins from the day an individual enters the organization. Newer members will commonly introduce and drive updated techniques and practices, such as ultrasound-guided regional anesthetic techniques. Individual physicians have the flexibility to plot a course to achieve their professional and financial goals.

Smaller anesthesiology practices can adhere to democratic practice governance. Practice leadership is often informal, and governance is a shared function among the organization's members. Governance models may be horizontally organized, promoting widespread input by practice members. Although the practice may be led by an elected president or governing body, the practicing members largely influence, or in extreme cases control, decisions of the practice. Many organizations seek to implement actions supported by member unanimity. Local, and less formal, governance provides the flexibility to make decisions collaboratively and instill new ideas quickly.

Small- to medium-sized private anesthesiology practices have the benefit of acting primarily for the benefit of their members. In the academic setting, anesthesiology represents 1 department among dozens of vertically integrated service lines. Anesthesiology departments can be negatively impacted by decisions benefiting the entire organization. To the contrary, independent small- and medium-sized anesthesia practices can identify and select practice opportunities aligned with their strategic goals.

Smaller practice physician anesthesiologists work with the surgeons as colleagues with the goals of providing the best, most time-effective and cost-efficient care possible. The ability to formally or informally consult and discuss care options benefits all involved. From the hospital leadership perspective, the ability to promptly address perioperative or anesthesiology-centric concerns is invaluable. In some instances, hospital leadership concerns mirror those of the anesthesiology practice. Leaders in smaller practices can work collaboratively with hospital leadership. Both organizations benefit through mutual understanding of the facility and its needs, and local understanding of the capabilities of the anesthesia group.

Limitations

Although small- to medium-sized anesthesia practice remains a prominent model of care, the legacy is challenged by the intricacies of an evolving medical landscape. As health care becomes more complex, anesthesiology practices have become increasingly driven to expand across sites, absorb other specialties, and grow within their health care system.

Financial incentives are declining for most medical specialties, including anesthesiology. In comparison with smaller practices, academic and large-anesthesiology practices can be sheltered from negative market forces. Many academic practices are vertically integrated across multiple medical specialties. This multispecialty construct provides a holistic approach to patient services and maximizes income across the practice. In addition, academic- and large-anesthesia practices benefit from nationally based third-party payer contracting. Small- to medium-sized practices often lack the network integration and buying power to compete with larger organizations.

Many small- to medium-sized practices are financially dependent on hospital contracts and stipends. This model has, in some settings, allowed smaller practices to maintain financial parity with larger groups. However, many hospitals are eliminating these contracts and remaining stipends or tying them to service and data-reporting requirements, which may be prohibitively onerous or expensive. Hospitals are financially driven to provide operating suite availability for their surgeons or proceduralists. The need for "on-demand" availability can operationally challenge smaller anesthesiology practices. Personnel requirements can evolve around contractually determined first starts, late operating suites, weekend operating suites, or procedural sites to meet the surgeons' preferences or hospital's strategic goals. From the anesthesiology practice perspective, this approach can result in staffing inefficiency, overhiring, limited scheduling flexibility, and reduced individual income.

Production pressure is a concern for many medical specialties, including anesthesiology. Small- to medium-sized anesthesia practices are especially vulnerable. The drive to satisfy contractual metrics and maintain efficiency can lead to an imbalance between production pressure and patient safety. In addition to contractual or financial components, the desire for anesthesiologists to maintain personal relationships with professional colleagues (eg, surgeons) can become an added driver. This pressure may lead to cutting corners on clinical care or safe staffing.

As previously stated, smaller practices can gain economic efficiencies by incrementally outsourcing operational services and reducing fixed overhead. However, increasing practice complexities are challenging this business model. Basic activities of sustaining a practice, such as billing and coding, require trained and experienced administrative staff. Additional personnel may be needed to manage compliance with federal and Joint Commission quality reporting requirements and to manage increased information technology scope and complexity. Although some of these services can be contracted from other businesses, outsourcing can limit control and oversight of basic but critical operational practice components.

other extreme, some large companies have invested heavily in optimizing information technology, HR management, quality improvement, and driving best clinical practice across multiple sites. Benefits and limitations of large-group practice are a function of their size, the distributed nature of their work, and the degree to which they are investing in the future.

Benefits

Large-group practices, by pooling resources, can make infrastructure investments that are beyond the reach of small groups and beyond the financial capabilities of academic departments. The return on these investments over time can lead to higher income for similar work. The obvious examples are the "back-office" functions of revenue cycle management, HR, payer contracting, and information technology. Anesthesia billing and collection is a complex business, uniquely different from other physician specialties, with a premium on specialty-specific expertise. Academic anesthesia groups often code cases, bill, and collect through a multispecialty physician practice plan or, worse, through the hospital system infrastructure. In the former case, there may be a lack of anesthesia-specific knowledge of optimal coding, billing, and collection strategies, whereas in the latter case, these shortcomings may be compounded by placing greater emphasis on negotiating contracts for hospital services rather than professional fees. Small private practices can purchase revenue cycle management services from anesthesia-specific practice management companies to avoid these pitfalls, but larger groups have the scope and scale to achieve even greater financial efficiency by bringing revenue cycle management in house.

Individual income in large groups can vary widely, depending on the specific model. At the low end, anesthesiologists are on salary (like in academic practices) with a relatively fixed return. At the high end, in partnership-model large groups, hard-working anesthesiologists can reap substantial returns: they profit both from their own work in a highly efficient organization and, if an equity holder, from the overall growth of the business. Their income is diversified across the entire scope of the business, such that loss of a local contract can be mitigated by success somewhere else. Understanding the compensation model and the potential for partnership should be important questions for prospective applicants.

Large groups typically maintain their own internal practice management mechanisms, including the components of revenue cycle management. Insourcing avoids the cost of outsourcing, of course, but has other benefits as well, including marginal gains in coding and collections based on specialty-specific expertise and incentivized focus on anesthesia. Large groups can invest more in the managed-care contracting game as well, by hiring sophisticated and experienced full-time negotiators. Achieving a few dollars more per unit in a given contract may not seem important but can add up rapidly; the largest large-group in America (US Anesthesia Partners) will bill for around 30 million units of anesthesia care in 2019. Some of the financial return is lost to clinicians because it is claimed by the business owners or financial investors in the large group, different from the incomes of academic programs or small groups, but a share of it remains at the local practice level; the net outcome is usually a gain for the clinician. Furthermore, greater financial returns can power greater investment in information technology, professional practice management services, and new growth, creating a self-sustaining virtuous cycle for sustained success.

HR management is necessary for any business, and an area where having the size to hire professionals can bring benefits to the group. Many desired HR benefits can be obtained at lower per-person costs when buying in quantity; this applies to generic items such as health care, dental insurance, and retirement plans as well as to specialty-specific items, such as malpractice insurance, anesthesia medications (eg, for office-based practice), and equipment. A higher level of HR expertise is additionally beneficial when difficult situations arise: for example, when there is a narcotic diversion event or an allegation of sexual harassment.

Large groups can invest more in comprehensive quality improvement programs. Investment in a quality improvement program has several benefits for members. First, it frees members of the group from having to learn the ever-changing landscape of federal regulatory requirements; this knowledge can be concentrated in just a few experts. Second, resources are available for supportive information technology, such as smartphone apps for quality and charge capture, automated patient satisfaction measurement, and regular feedback to clinicians. Finally, well-integrated large groups become a community of common interest for sharing best practices. A clinical "bright spot," such as a new enhanced recovery program, can be rapidly shared across the larger group. When clinicians at a single site encounter a clinical or practice management challenge, they can easily reach out for advice and resources from partners who have seen and surmounted a similar issue.

Although small groups benefit from close personal relationships among the partners, and can therefore make important decisions by consensus, large groups typically require more formal leadership structures. Defined local governance, with elected leadership and established term limits, mitigates the impact of idiosyncratic or tyrannical individuals, something that can warp the experience in small and academic groups. Large groups can invest in formal leadership training for their talented members; many also develop and promulgate career ladders that show new hires a clear pathway of promotion opportunities over time. In a climate where anesthesiology is a popular career, and is attracting the brightest and most ambitious medical students, this ability to promote leadership and career advancement opportunities is an important differentiator.

Large groups also have the ability to pool resources to increase their influence on the profession as a whole. Influence includes support for individuals in state and national leadership positions (eg, with the American Society of Anesthesiologists), support for participation with the American Board of

Anesthesiology, support for those in hospital leadership positions, and even support for political candidates. Filling these roles will have an influence on the future of the group itself, but also on the profession of anesthesiology. Because this kind of activity requires time out of the OR, large groups are better positioned to absorb the necessary loss of clinical revenue from individual leaders. Consistent with the other advantages of large-scale business, large anesthesia practices can devote more time, money, and expertise to state and national advocacy on key legislative issues. One of the exciting features of a large-group practice is the ability to positively influence the future, rather than just accept it as it arrives.

Limitations

There are limitations to practice in a large-group setting. Most important of these is loss of individual identity and autonomy at the local level. No one desires existence as just another cog in the machine, and no one wants Big Brother telling them how to practice. Assaying the internal culture of the group is thus a critical exercise for the aspiring member. Does the group really benefit from its size? Does it share a common vision, or is it just an amalgamation of diverse practices? Are individual clinicians treated like owners and partners or replaceable widgets? Who controls the care of patients? Are clinical decisions driven by local experts or by far-off businesspeople? Do clinicians value the resources they receive from the greater corporation, or is this benefit outweighed by the burden of increased bureaucracy?

As in private practice in general, large groups place a strong emphasis on clinical productivity. Potential hires should inquire carefully about the time and amount of work that will be required and should generally favor large groups that offer flexibility to meet their dynamic needs: premium income opportunities should be there for those who want to work extra hard, whereas arrangements for part-time and shared partnership should be there for those with family commitments or other external needs. A large group can also offer the flexibility to move geographically without having to start a career over.

The potential employee or partner should assess the motivation of anesthesiologists in the group. Are they engaged in making the practice better, or are they "locker-slammers" who just want to put in their 40 hours and go home? Small groups and academic practices may have an easier time building the right kind of engaged culture. Large groups can achieve this but face additional hurdles. One such hurdle is the potential conflict between the goals of the business (to return money to shareholders) and the goals of the individual (to provide excellent patient care in a stable long-term practice). Partnership model large groups have an easier time with this than publicly traded companies, but short-term financial goals may still trump long-term improvement. Another diversion of focus arises in the large anesthesia companies that include multiple other medical specialties. Are corporate decisions being made that favor anesthesiologists, or are they an afterthought behind emergency medicine or hospitalists or others?

Table 3
Benefits and risks of practice in a large, multisite anesthesia group

Pros	Cons
Greater income than academic practice; potential for entrepreneurial upside (depending on practice model)	Greater pressure for clinical productivity: greater time spent in direct patient care
Greater influence in the profession and greater external advocacy	Bureaucratic tendencies: slow to innovate, especially at the local level
More sophisticated infrastructure for revenue cycle management	Loss of motivation in salaried physicians with defined hours
More sophisticated infrastructure for regulatory reporting	Lack of alignment between business goals and patient care goals
Increased purchasing power for liability insurance, supplies, and HR benefits	Lack of single-specialty professional focus in multispecialty groups
Ability to share clinical information internally	Decreased local influence and focus if decisions are removed to a national structure
Ability to offer internal leadership training or sponsor external education	Lack of local control; economics may be harmed by events at distant sites
Better established and more transparent practice governance; less personality-based tyranny	
Clearly defined expectations at hiring; defined process for onboarding and career advancement	
Diversification or practice-based economic risk across multiple markets	
At larger scale can hire professional leadership for business functions: HR, billing and collection, contract negotiation, legal, and so forth	
Ability to scale across multiple specialties	

Summary: Large Group Practice

Large-group anesthesia practice has much to recommend it in terms of long-term stability, opportunities for personal growth, and financial returns; however, not all large anesthesia practices are the same. Table 3 summarizes the key benefits and limitations of this model of practice.

SUMMARY

Anesthesiology is a vibrant specialty with a bright future. Multiple practice models are available, distinguished by financial returns, entrepreneurial risk, governance structure, nonclinical support, and personal mission. The graduating resident or midcareer anesthesiologist contemplating a change of practice should consider the benefits and limitations of each model across multiple domains before choosing the model that will best advance their desired career.

References

[1] United States Bureau of Labor Statistics. Occupational employment statistics, 5/2018. Available at: https://www.bls.gov/oes/current/oes291061.htm#nat. Accessed April 30, 2019.
[2] Eichorn J. History of anesthesia patient safety. Int Anesthesiol Clin 2018;56(2):65–93.
[3] Institute of Medicine. To err is human. Washington, DC: National Academies Press; 2000. p. 144.
[4] Boggs SD, Barnett SR, Urman RD. The future of nonoperating room anesthesia in the 21st century: emphasis on quality and safety. Curr OpinAnaesthesiol 2017;30(6):644–51.
[5] Nagrebetsky A, Gabriel RA, Dutton RP, et al. Growth of nonoperating room anesthesia care in the United States. A contemporary trends analysis. Anesth Analg 2017;124(4):1261–7.
[6] Merrill DG. Value-based payment in ambulatory anesthesia: MACRA, MIPS, and more. Anesthesiol Clin 2019;37(2):373–88.
[7] American Society of Anesthesiologists 2018 Anesthesia Almanac. p. 78–9. Available at: https://www.asahq.org/research-and-publications/analytics-and-research-services. Accessed April 30, 2019.
[8] Frankl V. Man's search for meaning. Boston: Beacon Press; 1946.
[9] American Society of Anesthesiologists 2018 Anesthesia Almanac. Available at: https://www.asahq.org/research-and-publications/analytics-and-research-services. Accessed April 30, 2019.
[10] Available at: https://www.asahq.org/education-and-career/leadership-development. Accessed April 30, 2019.
[11] American Society of Anesthesiologists 2018 Anesthesia Almanac. p. 84–5. Available at: https://www.asahq.org/research-and-publications/analytics-and-research-services. Accessed April 30, 2019.

Advances in Anesthesia 37 (2019) 127–143

ADVANCES IN ANESTHESIA

Preoperative Patient Preparation, Programs, and Education in the United States

State of the Art, State of the Science, and State of Affairs

Solomon Aronson, MD, MBA, FCCP[a,*],
Mike P.W. Grocott, BSc, MBBS, MD, FRCA, FRCP, FFICM[b],
Michael (Monty) G. Mythen, MD[c]

[a]Anesthesiology and Population Health Science, Duke University School of Medicine, DUMC 3094, MS 33, 103 Baker House, Durham, NC 27710, USA; [b]University Southampton, University Road, South Hampton SO17 1BJ, UK; [c]University College London, 170 Tottenham Court Road, London W1T 7HA, UK

Keywords

• Perioperative medicine • Perioperative education • Preoperative assessment • Surgery

Key points

- We describe the state of the art for clinical preoperative patient preparation programs in the United States and give examples.
- We describe the state of the science for preoperative patient preparation process utilized in United States and United Kingdom and provide evidence to support best practice.
- We describe the state of the affairs for perioperative education in the United States and broader international Anesthesia community and provide examples of noteworthy programmatic education.

Statement of Commercial or Financial Conflicts and Funding Sources: S. Aronson, M.P.W. Grocott, M.G. Mythen have positions on the board of directors for the International Board of Perioperative Medicine (IBPOM). S. Aronson serves on the medical advisory board for Summus Global Inc. M.P.W. Grocott serves on the medical advisory board of Sphere Medical Ltd, NIHR Senior investigator. M.G. Mythen consults for Edwards life Sciences.

*Corresponding author. *E-mail address:* solomon.aronson@duke.edu

https://doi.org/10.1016/j.aan.2019.08.005

INTRODUCTION

Approximately 100,000 surgeries are performed in the United States each day and although perioperative complications affect relatively few of these patients, when complications do occur the management of these events consume a disproportional large amount of health care resources compared with costs of care for nonsurgical patients [1–5]. Although evidence strongly supports that the opportunity for greatest value enhancement in health care lies within the management of the most complex episodes of care for the sickest patients [6,7], one is left to wonder why preoperative patient preparation, albeit easy to rationalize [8–11], continues to have great variability of effectiveness and wide gaps in implementation. Emergencies and urgencies notwithstanding, the goal of preoperative preparation should be to reduce risk associated with surgery and facilitate functional recovery after surgery [12,13]. Despite these goals, variation in practice standards for determining a patient's readiness for surgery continues and the best approach for system integration and achieving surgical readiness (Box 1) is in an ongoing process.

Currently, most preoperative practice models (albeit not all) enable a preoperative history and examination, but do not proactively engage in closing gaps when preoperative patient surgical readiness is determined to be not optimal. The concept of a preanesthesia testing (PAT) clinic has become a threshold standard of a presurgical and preprocedural preparatory process. In this setting, patients are typically scheduled to have either an in-person clinic visit or a phone screen encounter determined by criteria depending on the originating surgical or procedural service [14]. Although an important goal of preoperative patient preparation is to prevent day-of-surgery case delays or cancellations, up to 20% of patients seen in a presurgical clinic have modifiable medical risks [15]. These modifiable risks are noted but likely not managed in a PAT model, whereby an appointment typically only enables a presurgery risk review, medication review, and presurgical history and physical examination

Box 1: Preoperative clinic organization tiers

Tier 1 - No formal preoperative clinic, pain service, or other hospital base structure

Tier 2 - Anesthesiology has formal relationship with a hospital base preoperative clinic

Tier 3- Anesthesiology manages preoperative assessment clinic and acute pain service

Tier 4 - Anesthesiology has comprehensive optimization, pain, and postoperative TOC services

Tier 5 – Above structured closely coordinated with institutional population health program(s)

Tier 6 – Above completely integrated within the health care system

Abbreviation: TOC, transition of care.

to be performed. This model may also allow for the anesthesia consent to be signed, the advance directive reviewed, and copays and other financial preparations to be completed. The request to schedule a PAT clinic visit, however, rarely occurs more than 30 days before the date of the procedure or surgery and commonly occurs only days before surgery. The timing of the PAT visit in this model provides minimal opportunity for effective preoperative patient preparation. By the time patients are scheduled to be seen in a preoperative clinic before an established surgery date, it is typically too late to modify their modifiable risk without an uneasy disruption of expectations. The preoperative physician is thus left with the dubious task of passing the risk information forward to the anesthesia and surgery care team. After risk stratification, the surgical care anesthesiologist is left to do the best she or he can under the circumstances. Because adverse outcomes occur infrequently and intraoperative management best efforts give a sense of contributing to an optimal result, we tend to underappreciate the impact of a forfeited opportunity to preoperatively shift the risk curve.

Ideally, the primary goal of preoperative patient preparation is to identify and reduce the risks associated with comorbid medical conditions affecting patients' perioperative outcomes. Additional goals would be to identify and initiate care to decrease the risk associated with common health issues of the perioperative patient independent of surgical intervention and to promote shared decision-making opportunities between patients, families, and provider for best course of action (which may include a decision not to undergo a surgery). Furthermore, confronting the need for surgery is an important teachable moment to influence long-term lifestyle change that is often underused [16]. Although there remains great variability among programs in their approach to preoperative patient preparation, herein are descriptions of the state of the science for preoperative patient preparation in the United States as well as some programs considered leading edge with respect to preoperative patient preparation process and programmatic education.

PREOPERATIVE PATIENT PREPARATION: STATE OF THE SCIENCE

Although every surgical procedure carries some degree of risk, this risk is usually relatively low. The risk for serious medical complications from surgery is less than 0.1% overall in healthy patients [17]. Healthy patients have significant physiologic reserves and tolerate major and minor surgical procedures well. The goal of preoperative patient preparation and risk assessment is to identify procedure- and patient-related factors that significantly increase the risk for complications at a cost in time and resources proportional to the risk.

Preoperative patient evaluation and preparation enables implementation of strategies to mitigate risk from the trauma of surgery. The normal biological and physiologic stress response of surgery is inflammation induced by cytokines released at the surgical site. This inflammatory cascade is accompanied by the release of endogenous hormones (eg, catecholamine) with the consequence of a hypercatabolic, procoagulation state with increased oxygen consumption, hyperglycemia, and intravascular fluid redistribution. That said, the specific type of surgery independently influences the risk for complications and also influences the risk for specific types of complications. Comorbid conditions such as heart disease, pulmonary disease, kidney and liver disease, diabetes mellitus, bleeding disorders, nutritional status, anemia, sleep apnea, smoking, hazardous alcohol use, and poor exercise tolerance also independently increase perioperative risk [18–22].

The evidence base for many preoperative interventions is in large part relatively poorly developed: a modest number of small, predominantly single-center studies are available to guide practice. As a consequence, few centers have implemented all the potentially beneficial interventions that are available to improve patient care before surgery. The 3 main categories of interventions are (i) shared decision making, (ii) comorbidity management, and (iii) prehabilitation. Critically important in enabling implementation for each of these areas is the so-called reengineering of the preoperative pathway [23,24].

Central to the definition of perioperative medicine is the temporal scope of interest: "from the moment of contemplation of surgery until full recovery" [25]. Recognition that the window of opportunity to intervene and benefit the patient opens at the moment that surgery is first contemplated is critical to effective implementation. A corollary to this observation is that the later the patient is engaged in the 3 core processes, the greater the lost opportunity to intervene and improve care. The moment of contemplation differs for different surgeries. For cancer surgery, it may be the moment the first screening test is completed (eg, cystoscopy, colonoscopy). For orthopedic surgery, the moment of contemplation is in the family doctor's office, in the physical therapist's office, or during a discussion with the surgeon. Moreover, although there is usually an urgency associated with major cancer surgery, owing to concerns about the clinical impact of disease progression if surgery is delayed, this is less likely to be the case for elective orthopedic surgery. Knee and hip replacement, the most common elective major orthopedic procedures, are undertaken with the aim of improving quality of life, rather than quantity. In this context, it is likely that the time taken to make considered shared decisions as well as to maximize the potential clinical benefits that may be achieved through comorbidity management and prehabilitation, will be time well spent.

An important feature of early engagement in the assessment and planning of perioperative care is that the processes of patient risk evaluation can occur in parallel with surgical assessment, rather than in series with it. Consequently, information obtained during the preoperative assessment can be fed into the surgical decision making process. In this way shared decision making [26,27] is facilitated and the so-called unnecessary surgery, where the risks of surgery outweigh the benefits, is less likely to happen. Where the preoperative assessment occurs later in the journey to surgery, it can be very difficult to reverse a settled surgical decision that the patient has become significantly invested in–

the opportunity for true shared decision making is at best diminished, and at worst lost.

Effective management of long-term conditions and acute illness is also more readily achieved when more time is available before surgery. Although comorbidity management has been a long-established component of preoperative assessment, early identification of pathology offers greater opportunity to intervene effectively. The most well-developed area in this regard is the management of preoperative anemia [28,29].

Anemia offers a relatively straightforward opportunity to improve care within a limited timeframe. There is a clearly defined and easily measurable abnormality, a noncomplicated diagnostic pathway, and a limited set of available management approaches that are typically rapidly effective at reversing the underlying abnormality. Hemoglobin levels obtained early in the pathway to surgery may be routinely screened by the perioperative team and abnormally low hemoglobin values may automatically trigger analysis of hematinic variables to categorize the type of anemia. For patients identified as iron deficient, iron therapy may be commenced by oral or intravenous routes depending on the severity of the abnormality and the proximity of the surgery. The value proposition for preoperative anemia is relatively straightforward owing to the consequent reduction in costs owing to reduced red blood cell transfusions [30].

Screening and optimization of cardiac, respiratory, and other comorbidities (malnutrition, diabetes, obstructive sleep apnea, pain, etc) often require more involved investigative routines but may still be governed by diagnostic and treatment algorithms.

Patients with poor glycemic control in the perioperative period or diagnosed diabetes often have serious comorbidities, such as cardiovascular disease, obesity, and chronic kidney disease, all of which significantly increase surgical risk [31]. Additionally, patients with diabetes undergoing surgery are more prone to postoperative infectious complications such as pneumonia, surgical site/wound infection, and sepsis [32,33], as well as longer hospital length of stays [34].

Obstructive sleep apnea occurs in approximately 20% of the population and is associated with serious perioperative complications, including cardiac arrhythmias, myocardial injury, and sudden death [35,36]. Patients who test positive for obstructive sleep apnea on screening should be referred for proper evaluation and management, as well as assessment for occult right heart failure. Postoperative airway adjuncts, such as continuous positive airway pressure, should be used when possible and appropriate.

The opportunity to improve patient care through prehabilitation–defined as intervention to enhance functional capacity in anticipation of a forthcoming physiologic stressor [37] may encompass behavioral change interventions including physical activity, exercise, diet and nutrition, and smoking and alcohol cessation strategies–is critically dependent on the amount of time available before surgery.

There is evidence that smoking and alcohol cessation before major surgery improves clinical outcomes, albeit in a limited number of small studies. Current

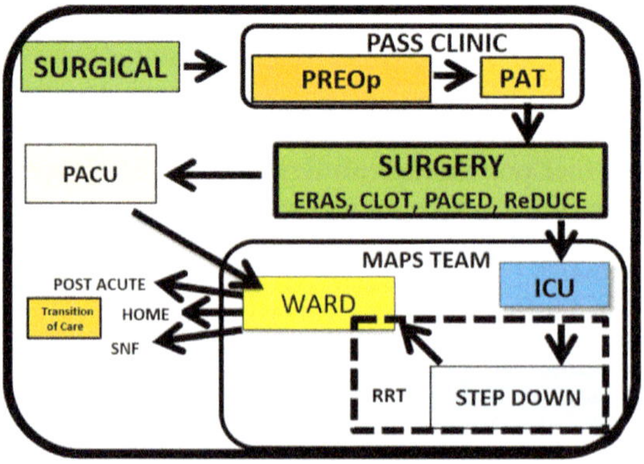

Fig. 1. The POET program. (*From* Aronson S, Westover J, Guinn N, et al. A Perioperative Medicine Model for Population Health: An Integrated Approach for an Evolving Clinical Science. Anesth Analg. 2018; 126(2): 682–90; with permission.)

a patient's status, calculate a score, and determine the threshold for phone or in-person visit criteria. If an in-person visit is deemed necessary, then a dedicated, physician led team of advanced practice providers focus attention to unique perioperative medical and social needs. The PASS clinic is a surgical care corridor whereby prescriptive preoperative screening, evaluation, and management of modifiable comorbid medical conditions occurs to enable and facilitate communication, education, medical management, surgical care coordination, and population health of at-risk patient populations. It also serves

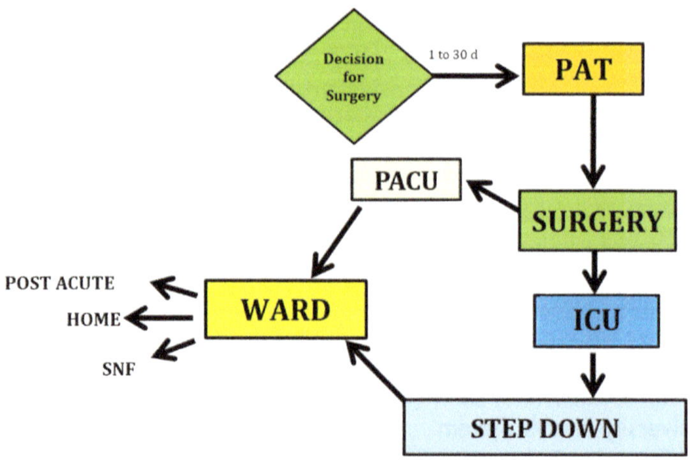

Fig. 2. Traditional pathway to surgery following declaration of surgery. (*From* Aronson S, Westover J, Guinn N, et al. A Perioperative Medicine Model for Population Health: An Integrated Approach for an Evolving Clinical Science. Anesth Analg. 2018; 126(2): 682–90; with permission.)

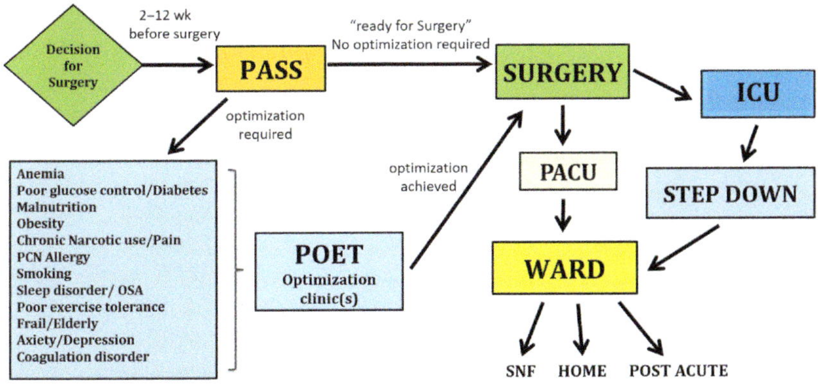

Fig. 3. PASS clinic pathway to surgery after declaration of surgery.

to increases alignment with best clinical practices and provide an important area for outcomes investigation. When referred to the PASS clinic, the patient's readiness for surgery is determined. After the evaluation, if further optimization of a modifiable condition is determined, then a referral to an optimization program is made.

The University of Michigan and Michigan Surgical and Health Optimization Program

The attending physicians review and supervise the assessment of every patient, order tests, write prescriptions and discuss issues with the primary care physicians and referring specialists as well as preform evaluations of consulted patients. A team of nurse practitioner, hospitalists and anesthesiologist performs the surgical history and physical examination as well as the anesthesiology assessments. Intrinsic to the University of Michigan's program is the Michigan Surgical and Health Optimization Program that analyzes surgical outcomes and their economic burden to insurance companies and payers. The program has identified preoperative exercise, nutrition, glucose control, pain management, deep venous thrombosis prophylaxis, obstructive sleep apnea screening, smoking cessation, and stress reduction strategies as directives to reduce cost and enhance value. A Centers for Medicare & Medicaid Services Innovation Grant among 40 hospitals between the Michigan Surgical Quality Collaborative, University of Michigan, and BCBS of Michigan has shown $2528 per case cost savings and 30% decreased hospital length of stay [61].

University of Texas at Austin, Dell Medical School

The Dell-Seton Preoperative ASSessment or Global Optimization (PASS-GO) Clinic has redefined its Pre-Admission Testing Clinic and has revised its name and focus. They use a system of risk stratification based on surgical procedure class and American Society of Anesthesiologists class to triage preoperative patient assessment toward a status of EXPRESS, PASS-GO. Regardless of triage status, evidence/consensus-based laboratory testing and diagnostic testing (when indicated) occurs. The PASS-GO clinic provides patient, family, and caregiver education and counseling; prehabilitation, including cardiopulmonary, nutritional, and psychological support; formal preoperative E/M consultation and intervention(s); and formal postdischarge transition care management [62].

The University of Texas MD Anderson Center

The PeriOperative Evaluation and Management Center (POEM) at MD Anderson performs comprehensive preoperative assessments to identify conditions that affect perioperative care. The clinic is staffed by a team of internists, anesthesiologists, advanced practice practitioners, nurses, and various clinic staff to evaluate patients following a determination for surgery. Patient chronic medical conditions and perioperative risks are identified and managed by anesthesiology and internal medicine. The POEM center offers support to help patients quit smoking, screens patients for obstructive sleep apnea, and provides penicillin allergy testing for patients with unconfirmed, self-reported allergies.

University of Washington: strong for surgery

Strong for Surgery is a presurgical health optimization program launched by the University of Washington for elective procedures. In 2016, the American College of Surgeons became the national home for Strong for Surgery. The American College of Surgeons has begun administering and promoting Strong for Surgery as a quality initiative aimed at identifying and evaluating evidence-based practices to optimize the health of patients before their operations. The aim of the program is to prepare patients for surgery by helping them become healthier. Patients are screened for several risk factors during a preoperative visit. Preoperative checklists, used to screen patients for risk factors that potentially could lead to surgical complications, provide guidance for interventions to help ensure better surgical outcomes. The checklists target 8 areas known to be highly influential determinants of surgical outcomes: medication management, nutrition, glycemic control, pain management, smoking cessation, delirium, prehabilitation, and patient directives.

PERIOPERATIVE EDUCATION: STATE OF AFFAIRS

In the specialty of anesthesiology, physicians must adapt to the changing clinical landscape surrounding surgical patient care. Perioperative medicine is an emerging subspecialty within anesthesiology that emphasizes the transition of care of patients from the time surgery is contemplated until full recovery. In recent years, there has been a trend toward new training and curricula that prepare the physician not merely for intraoperative care, but for the *entire continuum* of surgical care. As of 2018, 9 programs in the United States offered anesthesiology fellowships in perioperative medicine [63,64]. There is little published literature on perioperative care fellowship curricula, and current programs have a wide range of goals and teaching. The major traditional (non–Accreditation Council for Graduate Medical Education) perioperative fellowship programs in the United States are 1 year long and include several prestigious training programs (Table 1).

Table 1
Comparison of preoperative programs

Program	Core curriculum
Beth-Israel Deaconess	PSH/preoperative evaluation Leaderships Quality and safety Research/scholarship
Brigham & Women's	Preoperative evaluation OR management Quality and safety Geriatric, pain and palliative care Hospital leadership Innovation Ethics
Duke	Business operations/development Preoperative evaluation Perioperative risk stratification ERP Change management
Stanford	OR management Quality and safety Leadership Innovation
UC Irvine	Quality and safety Risk management Leadership Change management PSH and ERP OR Management Policy, ethics, biostatistics
UCLA	PSH, ERP Quality and safety Leadership Preoperative evaluation Population health
UCSD	OR management Preoperative management Executive leadership Pain/Regional management
University of Washington	Health economics Hospital management Quality and safety Health informatics
Vanderbilt	Preoperative evaluation Echo Perioperative consults

Abbreviations: ERP, enhanced recovery protocols; M&M, morbidity and mortality; MSc, masters of science; OR, operating room; POM, perioperative medicine; PSH, perioperative surgical home; QI, quality improvement.

In addition to traditional fellowship programs (albeit non–Accreditation Council for Graduate Medical Education), novel training curriculum and training options are being developed to deliver on meeting the unmet need for qualified individuals with enhanced training in perioperative medicine.

Morpheus fellowship

The Morpheus Consortium is an international collaboration between the Anesthesia Departments of Duke University in the United States and University College London and the University of Southampton in the UK. The Morpheus fellowship provides exposure to the science and implementation of perioperative medicine through online and in-person learning opportunities, by self-discovery and interaction with experts. It provides a unique on-line opportunity for anesthesia trainees who have the ambition of reaching outside of the operating room to gain practical, academic, clinical, operational, and research expertise in perioperative medicine. The curriculum is based around 3 key pillars: clinical care of patients; leadership and innovation including essential business skills, like operations, finance, communication; and leading change and the science of perioperative medicine. The primary online program allows a wide geographic dispersion of fellows in appropriate clinical facilities with on-site mentoring by associate faculty. It includes on-site travel to partner sites to observe effective delivery models in a range of health care systems and expected attendance at international conferences (eg, American Society of Anesthesiologists, Practice Management, Evidence Based Perioperative Medicine [EBPOM]) where they can attend curriculum specific state of the art sessions (discussed elsewhere in this article). Curriculum-specific conference content is also livestreamed where possible and recorded for secondary review with an on-line tutor or tutors to allow total participation.

International programs in perioperative management

Internationally, there has been formal recognition of the perioperative domain as unique and evolving for some time. The perioperative medicine programs around the world come in different guises and are led by a variety of clinicians (internists, anesthesiologists, nurses, advanced health providers, etc). There are, however, very few easily identifiable training standards or consistently structured and regulated training programs.

Among the most recognized international programs for perioperative medicine training are The University of Manitoba, The University of Toronto, The Alfred Hospital in Melbourne, Australia, The University of Australia, North Shore Hospital in Auckland, New Zealand, University College London, and the University of Southampton. Monash University, for example, in Melbourne, Australia, has been running perioperative medicine short courses and a masters in science for many years. The University College London has an online masters in science [65] and also runs an open source Massive Open On-line Course (MOOC) endorsed by the Royal College of Anaesthetists and The World Federation of Societies of Anesthesiologists [66]. To date, more than 15,000 people from more than 120 countries have taken the perioperative medicine MOOC. In January 2015, the Royal College of Anaesthetists launched its Perioperative Medicine Program endorsed by fellow Royal Colleges [67] and in June 2016 the UK General Medical Council approved a Curriculum amendment that included mandatory training in Perioperative Medicine to allow certification of completion of training in anesthesia (essential unit), thus setting a new standard [68]. In 2019, the Royal College of Anaesthetists have established a multiprofessional, multispecialty national Center for Perioperative Care in the UK to facilitate collaborative national initiatives for patient benefit. This center is a collaboration between the college and the Royal Colleges of Surgeons, Physicians, general practitioners (family doctors), and nursing along with patient and public representatives.

The International Board of Perioperative Medicine

Recently leaders in perioperative medicine from many of the institutions outside the United States and within the United States and other leaders from around the world have developed a perioperative medicine content outline and training curriculum to guide benchmarking and training in perioperative medicine. In the International Board of Perioperative Medicine training curriculum [69], the perioperative medicine learner would be expected to:

1. Demonstrate a patient centered approach to the integrative multidisciplinary care of patients contemplating or undergoing surgery.
2. Demonstrate expertise in the clinical management of patients in the perioperative period (ie, preoperative, intraoperative, acute postoperative, and postoperative transition of care periods).
3. Ensure that perioperative services are fully integrated, consistent, and reliable and make efficient use of resources.
4. Partner with colleagues in other disciplines, including primary care, surgeons, hospitalists, rehabilitation, geriatricians, nurses, and allied health professionals.
5. Demonstrate an advanced understanding of the importance and functioning of the preadmission process and/or clinic.
6. Educate the perioperative physician to risk stratify and optimize care of the patient in the perioperative period.
7. Develop the expertise to take a lead in collaborative decision making about the suitability of high risk patients for surgery.
8. Collaboratively manage the patient in the perioperative period, in particular high-risk surgical patients with acute or chronic medical comorbidities that require optimization and management to improve patient outcomes.
9. Obtain the managerial skills to lead a multidisciplinary perioperative management team.
10. Be equipped with research skills to understand perioperative medicine research.
11. Provide teaching to colleagues of all grades (levels) and specialties.

In addition to ongoing discussions to formalize perioperative medicine training curricula there are organizational efforts to share evidence and best practice information concerning the science of perioperative medicine.

[29] Meybohm P, Goehring MH, Choorapoikayil S, et al. Feasibility and efficiency of a preoperative anaemia walk-in clinic: secondary data from a prospective observational trial. Br J Anaesth 2017;118(4):625–6.

[30] Aleria Santini V, Truschi F, Bertelli A. Cost of red blood cell transfusion: an activity-based cost analysis. Blood 2010;116:3817.

[31] Golden SH, Peart–Vigilance C, Kao WH, et al. Perioperative glycemic control and the risk of infectious complications in a cohort of adults with diabetes. Diabetes Care 1999;22(9): 1408–14.

[32] Kalyani RR, Saudek CD, Brancati FL, et al. Association of diabetes, comorbidities, and A1C with functional disability in older adults: results from the National Health and Nutrition Examination Survey (NHANES), 1999–2006. Diabetes Care 2010;33(5):1055–60.

[33] Meneghini LF. Perioperative management of diabetes: translating evidence into practice. Cleve Clin J Med 2009;76(suppl 4):S53–9.

[34] Sharma A, Muir R, Johnston R, et al. Diabetes is predictive of longer hospital stay and increased rate of Clavien complications in spinal surgery in the UK. Ann R Coll Surg Engl 2013;95(4):275–9.

[35] Porhomayon J, Nader ND, Leissner KB, et al. Respiratory perioperative management of patients with obstructive sleep apnea. J Intensive Care Med 2014;29(3):145–53.

[36] Adesanya AO, Lee W, Greilich NB, et al. Perioperative management of obstructive sleep apnea. Chest 2010;138(6):1489–98.

[37] Levett DZH, Jack S, Grocott MPW. Fit for surgery? Perspectives on preoperative exercise testing and training.Richardson K. Br J Anaesth 2017;119(suppl_1):i34–43.

[38] Wong LS, Martins–Green M. Firsthand cigarette smoke alters fibroblast migration and survival: implications for impaired healing. Wound Repair Regen 2004;12(4):471–84.

[39] Barrera R, Shi W, Amar D, et al. Smoking and timing of cessation: impact on pulmonary complications after thoracotomy. Chest 2005;127(6):1977–83.

[40] Thomsen T, Villebro N, Møller AM. Interventions for preoperative smoking cessation. Cochrane Database Syst Rev 2014;(3):CD002294.

[41] Møller AM, Villebro N, Pedersen T, et al. Effect of preoperative smoking intervention on postoperative complications: a randomised clinical trial. Lancet 2002;359(9301):114–7.

[42] Eliasen M, Grønkjaer M, Skov–Ettrup LS, et al. Preoperative alcohol consumption and postoperative complications: a systematic review and meta–analysis. Ann Surg 2013;258(6): 930–42.

[43] Oppedal K, Møller AM, Pedersen B, et al. Pre-operative alcohol cessation prior to elective surgery. Cochrane Database Syst Rev 2012;(7):CD008343.

[44] Raebel MA, Newcomer SR, Reifler LM, et al. Chronic use of opioid medications before and after bariatric surgery. JAMA 2013;310(13):1369–76.

[45] Gan TJ, Robinson SB, Oderda GM, et al. Impact of postsurgical opioid use and ileus on economic outcomes in gastrointestinal surgeries. Curr Med Res Opin 2015;31(4):677–86.

[46] Oppeltz RF, Holloway TL, Covington CJ, et al. The contribution of opiate analgesics to the development of infectious complications in trauma patients. Int J Burns Trauma 2015;5(2):56–65.

[47] Carli F, Charlebois P, Stein B, et al. Randomized clinical trial of prehabilitation in colorectal surgery. Br J Surg 2010;97:1187–97.

[48] O'Doherty AF, West M, Jack S, et al. Preoperative aerobic exercise training in elective intracavity surgery: a systematic review. Br J Anaesth 2013;110(5):679–89.

[49] Sharma R, Ardebili MA, Abdulla IN. Does rehabilitation before total knee arthroplasty benefit postoperative recovery? A systematic review. Indian J Orthop 2019;53(1):138–47.

[50] McClave SA, Snider HL, Spain DA. Preoperative issues in clinical nutrition. Chest 1999;115(5 suppl):64S–70S.

[51] McClave SA, Martindale RG, Vanek VW, et al. Guidelines for the provision and assessment of nutrition support therapy in the adult critically ill patient: Society of Critical Care Medicine

(SCCM) and American Society for Parenteral and Enteral Nutrition (A.S.P.E.N.). JPEN J Parenter Enteral Nutr 2009;33(3):277–316.
[52] West MA, Wischmeyer PE, Grocott MPW. Prehabilitation and nutritional support to improve perioperative outcomes. Curr Anesthesiol Rep 2017;7(4):340–9.
[53] Jie B, Jiang ZM, Nolan MT, et al. Impact of preoperative nutritional support on clinical outcome in abdominal surgical patients at nutritional risk. Nutrition 2012;28(10):1022e7.
[54] Drover JW, Dhaliwal R, Weitzel L, et al. Perioperative use of arginine-supplemented diets: a systematic review of the evidence. J Am Coll Surg 2011;212(3):385–99, 99.e1.
[55] Burden S, Todd C, Hill J, et al. Pre-operative nutrition support in patients undergoing gastrointestinal surgery. Cochrane Database Syst Rev 2012;(11):CD008879.
[56] Levett DZH, Grimmett C. Psychological factors, prehabilitation and surgical outcomes: evidence and future directions. Anaesthesia 2019;74(Suppl 1):36–42.
[57] Li C, Carli F, Lee L, et al. Impact of a trimodal prehabilitation program on functional recovery after colorectal cancer surgery: a pilot study. Surg Endosc 2013;27(4):1072–82.
[58] Aronson S, Westover J, Guinn N, et al. A perioperative medicine model for population health: an integrated approach for an evolving clinical science. Anesth Analg 2018;126(2):682–90.
[59] Guinn NR, Hopkins TJ, Guercio JR, et al. Rational, development and implementation of a preoperative anemia clinic transfusion. Transfusion 2016;56:297–303.
[60] Setji T, Hopkins TJ, Jimenez M, et al, on behalf of the Duke Perioperative Enhancement Team (POET). Rationalization, development, and implementation of a preoperative diabetes optimization program designed to improve perioperative outcomes and reduce cost. Diabetes Spectr 2017;30(3):217–23.
[61] Englesbe MJ, Dimick JB, Sonnenday CJ, et al. The Michigan surgical quality collaborative: will a statewide quality improvement initiative pay for itself? Ann Surg 2007;246(6): 1100–3.
[62] Vetter TR, Uhler LM, Bozic KJ. Value-based healthcare: preoperative assessment and global optimization (PASS-GO): improving value in total joint replacement care. Clin Orthop Relat Res 2017;475(8):1958–62.
[63] Gharapetian A, Chung F, Wong D, et al. Perioperative fellowship curricula in anesthesiology: a systematic review. Can J Anesth 2015;62:403–12.
[64] Koepke E, Williams DGA. Perioperative medicine: a new subspecialty, or the future of anesthesia? ASA Monitor 2018;82:68–9.
[65] Available at: https://www.ucl.ac.uk/prospective-students/graduate/taught-degrees/perioperative-medicine-msc. Accessed September 25, 2019.
[66] Available at: https://www.futurelearn.com/courses/perioperative-medicine. Accessed September 25, 2019.
[67] Available at: https://www.rcoa.ac.uk/perioperativemedicine. Accessed September 25, 2019.
[68] Available at: https://www.rcoa.ac.uk/CCT/AnnexD. Accessed September 25, 2019.
[69] Available at: http://www.internationalboardpom.org. Accessed September 25, 2019.
[70] Ryan SP, Howell CB, Wellman SS, et al. Pre-operative optimization checklists within the CJR bundle have not decreased hospital returns for total knee arthroplasty. J Arthroplasty 2019;34(7S):S108–13.
[71] Bernstein DN, Liu TC, Winegar AL, et al. Evaluation of a preoperative optimization protocol for primary hip and knee arthroplasty patients. J Arthroplasty 2018;(33):3642–8.

Advances in Anesthesia 37 (2019) 145–162

ADVANCES IN ANESTHESIA

ELSEVIER
MOSBY

Anesthesia Informatics in 2018

Allan F. Simpao, MD, MBI[a,*],
Mohamed A. Rehman, MD[b]

[a]Department of Anesthesiology and Critical Care, University of Pennsylvania Perelman School of Medicine, Children's Hospital of Philadelphia, 3401 Civic Center Blvd., Philadelphia, PA 19104, USA; [b]Department of Anesthesiology, Johns Hopkins All Children's Hospital, 501 6th Avenue South, St Petersburg, FL 33701, USA

Keywords

• Anesthesia • Information management • Perioperative • Decision support • Database • Electronic health record • Quality improvement • Research

Key points

- Anesthesiologists, other clinicians, and researchers have long endeavored to derive meaningful insights from data captured by electronic health record and anesthesia information management systems to achieve myriad goals: improving patient care, researching perioperative outcomes, enhancing financial oversight and responsibility, and many others.
- Clinical informatics is the application of clinical data to improve health care processes and systems, and anesthesia informatics is a subset of clinical informatics that encompasses the application of informatics to perioperative and anesthesia data.
- This narrative review describes the state of anesthesia informatics in 2018, the historical developments leading to the current state, and potential future applications of informatics in anesthesia care.

INTRODUCTION

Technology is present throughout contemporary anesthesia practice. Vital sign monitors and anesthesia machines capture physiologic and ventilator data that are both immediately available on the devices and transmitted to electronic health record (EHR) systems and anesthesia information management systems, thereby eliminating the need for paper charting. Anesthesiologists, other clinicians, and researchers have endeavored to derive meaningful insights from

Disclosures: The authors have nothing to disclose.

*Corresponding author. *E-mail address:* simpaoa@email.chop.edu

https://doi.org/10.1016/j.aan.2019.08.006

these data with the goals of improving patient care, researching perioperative outcomes, enhancing financial oversight and responsibility, and many others. Clinical informatics is the application of clinical data to improve health care processes and systems, and anesthesia informatics is a subset of clinical informatics that encompasses the application of informatics to perioperative and anesthesia data.

This narrative review describes the state of anesthesia informatics in 2018, the historical developments leading to the current state, and potential future applications of informatics in anesthesia care. The review begins with an overview of clinical and anesthesia informatics, followed by a section on anesthesia information management systems, anesthesia documentation integrated in EHR systems, and clinical decision support (CDS). It next describes secondary uses of anesthesia data and methods by which these data can be mined and analyzed, and goes on to discuss future directions and possibilities.

AN OVERVIEW OF CLINICAL AND ANESTHESIA INFORMATICS FROM THE 1990S TO 2018

Although microcomputers were used routinely in hospitals in the 1990s, it was not until a decade later that initiatives to harness computer and information technology to improve health care became more widespread. Advances in computer and networking technology, patient monitoring systems, and EHR systems enabled hospitals to accumulate a rapidly increasing volume and widening variety of patient data [1,2]. In 2009, the United States Federal Government enacted the Health Information Technology for Economic and Clinical Health (HITECH) Act, which incentivized health care institutions and providers to implement EHRs to enhance the quality and efficiency of health care [3]. EHRs collect patient care data in electronic form that can be explored and analyzed for many purposes, including improving patient care, optimizing resource use, and informing decision making at the clinical and enterprise levels [4].

The pursuit of these goals created an increasing demand for clinicians trained in informatics who were well versed in both the medical and information sciences [5]. In 2007, the American Medical Informatics Association (AMIA) began to develop the core content and training requirements for a subspecialty of clinical informatics because they recognized the unique role that informatics-trained physicians could serve in the setting of the ongoing convergence of the computer and information sciences with health care. AMIA led the establishment of professional-level education and certification for physicians in informatics, which resulted in clinical informatics as a board-certified medical subspecialty under the American Board of Preventive Medicine [6]. Clinical informatics is situated at the convergence between the information and medical sciences, and has been defined as "a body of knowledge, methods, and theories that focus on the effective use of information and knowledge to improve the quality, safety, and cost-effectiveness of patient care as well as the health of both individuals and populations." [3] Clinical informatics covers a wide array of topics, including electronic clinical documentation, computerized provider order entry systems, and CDS, and ongoing developments in computational power, database management, physiologic monitoring devices, and software applications have set the stage for increasingly sophisticated data analytics and informatics applications in clinical care.

Anesthesia informatics consists of the myriad applications of clinical informatics and the use of EHR and perioperative data to derive meaningful clinical insights and improve anesthesia and perioperative care [7]. Anesthesiologists are included in the growing group of physicians who have obtained expertise and board certification in clinical informatics, and certification involves both a firm understanding of the hardware and software that comprise hospital systems and familiarity with team management strategies and development methodologies [8]. An ever-growing number of anesthesiologists and other health care providers interact with EHRs and other technology on a daily basis. Anesthesia informatics harnesses this interaction and focuses on using information systems to optimize workflow, enable research studies of perioperative physiology on a large scale, and acquire a better understanding of the quality of anesthesia care as well as the outcomes of patients who undergo anesthesia and surgery [8].

Of the 36 physicians who were board certified in both anesthesiology and clinical informatics as of January 1, 2016, most were satisfied with the clinical informatics boards, and most stated that informatics expertise was important to anesthesiology [9]. More than 75% of the anesthesiologist-informaticians held a role in the hospital outside of their anesthesiology departments; these institutional roles are part of what makes clinical informatics so crucial to the future of anesthesiology [8,9]. Until 2022, physicians can obtain certification by spending at least 10 h/wk practicing medical informatics for 3 years (the practice pathway) or by completing a 24-month Accreditation Council for Graduate Medical Education (ACGME)–accredited fellowship in clinical informatics. After 2022, the practice pathway will end, and the only path to certification will be via the fellowship pathway. The respondents were skeptical that anesthesiology residents would elect to complete a 24-month ACGME fellowship in clinical informatics in order to sit for the certification examination [9]. As of 2018, there were approximately 50 individuals who were board certified in anesthesiology and clinical informatics, which constitutes only approximately 0.1% of the more than 53,000 board-certified anesthesiologists in the United States [8].

Before delving into the nuances and many examples of applications of anesthesia informatics, it is important to understand the collection of perioperative data via electronic means. Thus, the evolution of the anesthesia record from paper charting to current electronic methods is discussed next. Anesthesia information management systems (AIMSs) are either integrated components of the EHR or stand-alone software and hardware products that were developed as a means to document the details of an anesthetic and the patient's physiologic status while receiving anesthesia. AIMSs and integrated EHRs are defined long-term effects of such a mandatory quality assurance reporting system for adverse events at 2 academic medical centers found a decrease in preventable intraoperative adverse events [21].

Integrated EHRs and stand-alone AIMSs are used currently not only throughout traditional operating room perioperative care but also wherever anesthesia care is provided both inside and outside of the hospital [22]. This system includes documentation of acute pain services and recommendations as well as the delivery of anesthesia on the labor and delivery unit and during ICU bedside procedures [23,24].

Successful AIMS and integrated EHR implementations as well as transitions from AIMSs to integrated EHRs require substantial investments in hardware, software, and so-called peopleware; that is, clinicians such as anesthesiologist-informaticians with the necessary informatics expertise to lead the decision-making and implementation processes [8,18]. Financial costs for implementations and transitions obviously vary depending on the hardware and software required for the chosen level of sophistication and, most importantly, the lost clinical productivity of the implementation team as clinicians' time is dedicated to site visits, meetings, and other activities [18]. Note that an AIMS is not a one-off purchase but requires an ongoing commitment to technical support and software updates to keep the AIMS current and functional.

Capture and storage of the diverse mix of data via stand-alone AIMSs and integrated EHRs depends on the monitoring devices, computer hardware, and data and networking infrastructure. Typical AIMS and integrated EHR hardware components include a computer workstation and either mounting equipment to affix the computer to the anesthesia machine or a wheeled mobile stand, and devices such as special keyboards, bar code scanners, or syringe pumps may also be included [23]. Compatible physiologic device interfaces are essential to allow patient physiologic monitors, anesthesia machines, ventilators, and other monitors to communicate and record automatically via the AIMS or integrated EHR hardware and software [23]. Stand-alone AIMS software on a workstation is typically in the form of a so-called thick client that stores the anesthesia data on that workstation; the data are then filed periodically to a central server. With integrated EHRs, the software on the computer workstation displays a user interface referred to as a thin client, with most or all of the data filed directly to a central server [18,23]. The physiologic monitor and anesthesia machine data flow from the devices to the client and then the server, or first to the server and then the client workstations, depending on the setup. In some implementations, the physiologic device data flow to the AIMS or integrated EHR through a separate medical device integration interface (also known as middleware) that offers additional functionality such as higher-fidelity data sampling [25]. It is important to keep in mind any disparities in data sampling rates when analyzing data from both the middleware device and the AIMS or EHR, because events such as hypoxemia may look drastically different based on data granularity [26]. For example, a 15-minute rolling average of heart rate might miss the changes associated with a sudden dysrhythmia that can only be seen in the data when granularity is at the single-second level.

Box 1 lists some of the domains in which stand-alone AIMSs were shown to provide positive benefits to patients, clinicians, and hospitals [27]. Anesthesia

Box 1: Benefits of anesthesia information management systems published in peer-reviewed literature

Improved patient safety and quality of care

- Anesthesia care team does not have to spend time manually recording vital signs
- Enable automated systems to perform drug diversion surveillance
- Provide automatic notification of operating room location errors
- Warn users of potential drug allergy and blood transfusion reactions
- Facilitate implementation of and adherence to departmental protocols, such as perioperative antibiotic prophylaxis administration
- Provide point-of-care clinical decision support, such as perioperative glucose management
- Enable real-time surveillance of patient monitors
- Provide timely post hoc reports via e-mail or text messaging to affect clinicians' behavior

Improved documentation

- Precise, accurate capture of perioperative data and patients' anesthetic details
- Generate high-resolution anesthetic records that are more easily searched, accessed, and used for secondary use than paper records
- Automated, real-time, or near-real-time notification of missing or incomplete documentation
- Facilitate risk management and quality assurance activities

Improved operations management

- Improve billing personnel work flow when reviewing anesthesia records
- Enhance anesthesiology department's administrative role in the perioperative setting
- Facilitate faculty and staff scheduling
- Generate a real-time surgical whiteboard to improve situational awareness and workflow
- Enable operating room modeling for administrative decision support
- Facilitates individual anesthesia provider and departmental performance tracking
- Allows verification of ACGME case requirements for residents and fellows
- Provide post hoc reports to residents with a log of their anesthesia experiences to guide requests for next day's cases

AIMS [39,55]. Anesthesia departments and practices that transition from legacy AIMSs to integrated EHRs must either attempt to replicate their CDS tools using the alerts and other features available in the EHR system or abandon them. Another option is to use software systems that can run concurrently with the EHR to provide integration of patient data streams and provide CDS functionality. AlertWatch (Ann Arbor, MI) is one such CDS monitoring system that integrates aggregated data from physiologic monitors and the EHR and presents CDS alerts to clinicians [56,57]. The system has been used to manage intraoperative hyperglycemia and to generate automated alerts on the labor and delivery floor [58,59]. AlertWatch was also shown to improve process measures, but not postoperative clinical outcomes, in a recent 6-year study [60].

Research and innovations in anesthesia CDS are ongoing in 2018. The evidence for near-real-time, point-of-care CDS in anesthesia remains promising, albeit limited, despite the proliferation of AIMS in US academic anesthesia departments, with an approximately 84% adoption rate anticipated between 2018 and 2020 [61]. Although the necessary skill and experience to develop research platforms for CDS may not be widely disseminated among anesthesiology practices, one solution may be for anesthesia departments to include more clinical informatics training for trainees [39]. The paucity of near-real-time, point-of-care anesthesia CDS articles may also be caused by the challenges associated with conducting and publishing these studies, and the ongoing transition to integrated EHRs carries the risk of limiting the ability for anesthesia informatics professionals to implement, support, and track CDS tools [39]. However, one benefit to the transition to integrated EHRs is the potential to more easily conduct multicenter studies of CDS tools, because anesthesia departments and practices may have the option to share their CDS implementations with others who are using the same EHR.

Anesthesia CDS is a dynamic and innovative field that is likely to remain an active area of anesthesia informatics research in the near future. Despite the challenges that are associated with conducting studies of anesthesia CDS, such research is necessary to enhance patient safety, improve understanding of which CDS tools are effective, and ensure that CDS development and implementation in anesthesia are based on high-quality evidence from multiple centers.

SECONDARY USES OF ANESTHESIA INFORMATION MANAGEMENT SYSTEM AND ELECTRONIC HEALTH RECORD DATA

Countless institutions, anesthesia practices, and individuals have used AIMS and EHR data that have been collected during the daily process of patient care for various purposes, including clinical research, quality improvement, and collaborative initiatives [62]. Data validity is of great importance, because the quality and reliability of manually entered data in the AIMS or integrated EHR often depend on the users [63,64]. Furthermore, physiologic data that are captured by the AIMS and EHR also have inherent artifacts that must be considered [65,66]. Research, quality improvement initiatives, and other efforts that rely on anesthesia data must take into account these artifacts to avoid faulty conclusions referred to colloquially as garbage in, garbage out [67]. Clear, consistent definitions of perioperative events and outcomes facilitate valid, reliable documentation; these definitions routinely vary across, and sometimes even within, institutions [18,68]. Anesthesia departments and practices that have migrated from an AIMS to an integrated EHR must also deal with the issue of storing data from the older legacy system in a separate perioperative data "warehouse" if the data are to be used for secondary purposes, because EHRs are typically not designed to store and make the legacy data easily available to users [69]. Data warehouses can also be used to make AIMS data more easily accessible for secondary purposes that might otherwise be difficult to obtain directly from the EHR [70].

One popular and current use of AIMS and EHR data is to combine data from multiple institutions in collaborative data registries to create larger data pools to study rare events or outcomes, or patients with rare diseases or conditions. Many studies have been published in the years up to and including 2018 using data from multicenter anesthesia registries such as the Multicenter Perioperative Outcomes Group and the Anesthesia Quality Institute's National Anesthesia Clinical Outcomes Registry [71,72]. Collaborative data registry efforts such as Wake Up Safe, the Pediatric Craniofacial Collaborative Group, and the Pediatric Difficult Intubation Registry have also recently produced meaningful insights in pediatric anesthesia regarding medication errors, craniofacial cases, and pediatric difficult airway management [73–75]. There are myriad other examples of recently published research studies based on registry data. Although reporting outcomes data can be a sensitive topic among clinicians and anesthesia practices, participation in a collaborative registry allows benchmarking of performance against other providers and practices and enables researchers to conduct novel and generalizable studies using larger datasets [76].

Anesthesia registries are a thriving area of anesthesia informatics and will continue to proliferate, recruit contributors, and increase in size, creating a greater pool of collaborative data for data mining and research. Initiatives such as the US Meaningful Use program will continue to incentivize aggregation of data at a national level through health information exchanges and national repositories [77]. Efforts by the federal government should increase the interoperability and data-sharing capabilities across various EHRs, further fueling the contribution of data to these large anesthesia data collaborations.

ANALYTICAL APPROACHES TO ANESTHESIA INFORMATION MANAGEMENT SYSTEM AND ELECTRONIC HEALTH RECORD DATA

Large anesthesia datasets can arise not only from multicenter collaborative efforts but also from mining a single institution's perioperative vital sign and medication data. Advanced analytical methods offer one solution to managing such voluminous and diverse datasets. One such approach is visual analytics, which is defined as the science of analytical reasoning facilitated by interactive visual interfaces. Visual analytics has been used to enhance the evaluation of large, complex datasets within health care [66]. Visual analytics tools are computational software that integrate data analytics with interactive visual interfaces and can be used to navigate and manipulate large datasets [4]. These tools enable users to create dashboards that display histograms and graphs in order to identify data trends. However, proper visual analytics techniques require more than haphazardly arraying graphs and buttons across a display; fundamental principles for effective visual analytics dashboard design include displaying critical information on a single screen while minimizing the object clutter, sparse use of graphical icons, abbreviating displayed context, and using graded color intensities rather than a clashing mix of hues [78].

The data are stored in a dimensional database model rather than a traditional relational database model to facilitate data querying and analysis on a large scale. Dimensional models are implemented using online analytical processing systems that were developed specifically to analyze very large datasets. Dimensional models create a fact table that contains all of the potential data transactions as well as filters (dimensions) around the table that will be used to associate facts and measures throughout the dimensional database. This system results in simplified querying scripts with execution durations that are significantly briefer than those of the more complex relational model scripts [4,79].

After the data have been audited, validated, and stored in a dimensional database, visual analytics tools are used to construct user-friendly dashboards that display histograms and graphs in order to identify and explore data trends. Visual analytics tools enable exploration and hypothesis generation in large datasets, and empower users to access the data in a way that facilitates understanding [68]. Data elements of interest can be tracked over time to assess their appropriateness and proper use, and filters can be applied to visualize trends and patterns. Point-and-click functionality allows the user to access the data, often in near real time, for periodic assessment of progress.

Visual analytics tools have been applied in various ways to anesthesia data in recent years. Researchers have used visual analytics to quickly determine the use of preoperative anesthesia assessments [80]. Perioperative transfusion practice has been analyzed across approximately 230,000 anesthetic records using visual analytics software, and this information has been used to guide policies for ordering blood products [81]. Visual analytics software has also been used to compute millions of data points comprising vital signs, end-tidal volatile agent, end-tidal carbon dioxide, and many other data points across 15 years of anesthetics in infants undergoing surgery [82].

Visual analytics facilitates investigative analysis by showing connections between entities and focusing on essential information [83]. Thus, data exploration using visual analytics can guide the selection and application of other advanced analytics techniques and methods. Visual analytics works well as a tool to engage in descriptive analytics, which involves deriving meaningful insight from data. This type of analysis is retrospective (ie, showing what has happened), whereas predictive analytics involves mining data to predict an outcome (ie, what will happen).

Machine learning is an advanced analytics technique that involves using computer algorithms that can discover associations in large datasets in a supervised or unsupervised fashion. Although traditional statistical methods such as logistic models can predict postoperative outcomes with a high degree of accuracy, there is a growing movement among anesthesia informatics researchers to apply machine learning algorithms to large, diverse AIMS and EHR datasets for predictive analytics [84]. Many examples of machine learning being applied to perioperative and anesthesia data were published in 2017 and 2018: defining and predicting pain volatility in users of a pain management app [85], improving the efficiency of the operating room environment [86], predicting postinduction hypotension [87], modeling postintubation hypoxia [88], predicting periventricular leukomalacia in neonates after cardiac surgery [89], detecting airway management technique in anesthesia records [90], predicting postoperative in-hospital mortality [91], and predicting hypotension based on arterial pressure waveforms [92].

This small sample is only a few of the applications of machine learning in anesthesia informatics over a 2-year period. The complexity and size of large anesthesia and perioperative datasets are clearly fertile ground for machine learning algorithms to be designed and used to derive meaningful information and provide predictive analytics. Anesthesiologist-informaticians who are well versed in advanced analytics methods or who have teams with advanced analytics experts are poised ideally for the current increasing trend of machine learning in anesthesia informatics.

THE FUTURE OF ANESTHESIA INFORMATICS

This review is not intended to be an exhaustive description of the ongoing convergence of information technology and anesthesiology. As stand-alone AIMSs continue to give way to integrated EHRs, anesthesia modules in EHRs should continue to advance in use and functionality, and automated data capture will be made possible from a growing array of devices, such as barcode medication labeling systems and smart medication infusion pumps [93,94]. Analytical techniques such as machine learning and visual analytics will enable descriptive and predictive analytics of large anesthesia datasets and perioperative data warehouses [4]. Machine learning algorithms will also be applied to anesthesia data to automate perioperative event capture and derive clinical meaning from, or assign clinical relevance to, physiologic data. Real-time analysis of patient data across disparate health information systems through the use of sophisticated CDS and surveillance systems is another promising application of technology to anesthesia data [95]. AIMS-based and EHR-based CDS will continue to be developed in more sophisticated and meaningful ways to enhance various facets of patient care, and interoperability across different software platforms will facilitate data sharing across practices and institutions. The rapid pace of development of informatics tools and sophisticated monitoring equipment will help to unlock the potential of analytics combined with genomics and real-time CDS to optimize the care of patients [96].

References

[1] Wolfe PJ. Making sense of big data. Proc Natl Acad Sci U S A 2013;110:18031–2.
[2] Costa FF. Big data in biomedicine. Drug Discov Today 2014;19:433–40.
[3] Stark P. Congressional intent for the HITECH act. Am J Manag Care 2010;16:24–8.
[4] Simpao AF, Ahumada LM, Rehman MA. Big data and visual analytics in anaesthesia and health care. Br J Anesth 2015;115(3):350–6.
[5] Detmer DE, Shortliffe EH. Clinical informatics: prospects for a new medical subspecialty. JAMA 2014;311:2067–8.
[6] Shortliffe EH. President's column: subspecialty certification in clinical informatics. J Am Med Inform Assoc 2011;18:890–1.
[7] Stabile M, Cooper L. Review article: the evolving role of information technology in perioperative patient safety. Can J Anaesth 2013;60:119–26.
[8] Hofer IS, Levin MA, Simpao AF, et al. Anesthesia informatics grows up. Anesth Analg 2018;127(1):18–20.
[9] Poterack KA, Epstein RH, Dexter F. The anesthesiologist-informatician: a survey of physicians board-certified in both anesthesiology and clinical informatics. Anesth Analg 2018;127(1):115–7.
[10] Klar R. Selected impressions on the beginning of the electronic medical record and patient information. Methods Inf Med 2004;43:537–42.
[11] Wright AJ. Early use of the Cushing-Codman anesthesia record. Anesthesiology 1987;66: 92.
[12] Lerou JG, Dirksen R, van Daele M, et al. Automated charting of physiological variables in anesthesia: a quantitative comparison of automated versus handwritten anesthesia records. J Clin Monit 1988;4:37–47.
[13] Gravenstein JS. The uses of the anesthesia record. J Clin Monit 1989;5:256–65.
[14] Peters RM. Interactive microcomputer for acquisition of patient information. J Clin Monit 1989;5:266–9.
[15] Monica K. Most significant Epic, Cerner health IT achievements of 2017. Available at: https://ehrintelligence.com/news/most-significant-epic-cerner-health-it-achievements-of-2017. Accessed April 24, 2019.
[16] Ehrenfeld JM, Rehman MA. Anesthesia information management systems: a review of functionality and installation considerations. J Clin Monit Comput 2011;25:71–9.
[17] Kadry B, Feaster WW, Macario A, et al. Anesthesia information management systems: past, present, and future of anesthesia records. Mt Sinai J Med 2012;79:154–65.
[18] Simpao AF, Rehman MA. Anesthesia information management systems. Anesth Analg 2018;127:80–94.
[19] Epstein RH, Dexter F, Schwenk ES. Provider access to legacy electronic anesthesia records following implementation of an electronic health record system. J Med Syst 2019;43(5): 105.
[20] Peterfreund RA, Driscoll WD, Walsh JL, et al. Evaluation of a mandatory quality assurance data capture in anesthesia: a secure electronic system to capture quality assurance information linked to an automated anesthesia record. Anesth Analg 2011;112:1218–25.
[21] Wanderer JP, Gratch DM, Jacques PS, et al. Trends in the prevalence of intraoperative adverse events at two academic hospitals after implementation of a mandatory reporting system. Anesth Analg 2018;126:134–40.
[22] Bouhenguel JT, Preiss DA, Urman RD. Implementation and use of anesthesia information management systems for non-operating room locations. Anesthesiol Clin 2017;35: 583–90.

[23] Shah NJ, Tremper KK, Kheterpal S. Anatomy of an anesthesia information management system. Anesthesiol Clin 2011;29:355–65.
[24] Simpao AF, Galvez JA, England WR, et al. A technical evaluation of wireless connectivity from patient monitors to an anesthesia information management system during intensive care unit surgery. Anesth Analg 2016;122:425–9.
[25] Zaleski J. Medical device integration: a world of possibilities. Available at: https://www.mddionline.com/medical-device-integration-world-possibilities. Accessed April 25, 2019.
[26] Simpao AF, Ma AA, Tan JM, et al. One laryngospasm, 2 realities: a case report highlighting the impact of data granularity on post hoc analysis of perioperative events. A A Pract 2018;11(11):315–7.
[27] Simpao AF, Ehrenfeld JM. Special case: perioperative information management systems. In: Ehrenfeld JM, Cannesson M, editors. Monitoring technologies in acute care environments. New York: Springer Verlag; 2014. p. 391–7.
[28] Gardner RM, Prakash O. Challenges and opportunities for computerizing the anesthesia record. J Clin Anesth 1994;6(4):6333–41.
[29] Bloomfield EL, Feinglass NG. The anesthesia information management system for electronic documentation: what are we waiting for? J Anesth 2008;22:404–11.
[30] Thrush DN. Are automated anesthesia records better? J Clin Anesth 1992;4:386–9.
[31] Reich DL, Wood RK Jr, Mattar R, et al. Arterial blood pressure and heart rate discrepancies between handwritten and computerized anesthesia records. Anesth Analg 2000;91:612–6.
[32] O'Sullivan CT, Dexter F, Lubarsky DA, et al. Evidence-based management assessment of return on investment from anesthesia information management systems. AANA J 2007;75(1):43–8.
[33] Davis TC, Green JA, Colquhoun A, et al. Anesthesia recordkeeping: accuracy of recall with computerized and manual entry recordkeeping. J Clin Monit Comput 2012;26:163–9.
[34] Feldman JM. Do anesthesia information systems increase malpractice exposure? Results of a survey. Anesth Analg 2004;99:840–3.
[35] Hunt DL, Haynes RB, Hanna SE, et al. Effects of computer-based clinical decision support systems on physician performance and patient outcomes: a systematic review. JAMA 1998;280:1339–46.
[36] Shortliffe EH. Medical informatics and clinical decision making: the science and the pragmatics. Med Decis Making 1991;11:S2–14.
[37] Osheroff JA. Improving medication use and outcomes with clinical decision support: a step-by-step guide. Chicago: The Healthcare Information and Management Systems Society; 2009.
[38] Simpao AF, Tan JM, Lingappan AM, et al. A systematic review of near real-time and point-of-care clinical decision support in anesthesia information management systems. J Clin Monit Comput 2017;31:885–94.
[39] Freundlich RE, Ehrenfeld JM. Anesthesia information management: clinical decision support. Curr Opin Anaesthesiol 2017;30(6):705–9.
[40] Nair BG, Gabel E, Hofer I, et al. Intraoperative clinical decision support for anesthesia: a narrative review of available systems. Anesth Analg 2017;124:603–17.
[41] Epstein RH, Dexter F, Patel N. Influencing anesthesia provider behavior using anesthesia information management system data for near real-time alerts and post hoc reports. Anesth Analg 2015;121:678–92.
[42] Chau A, Ehrenfeld JM. Using real-time clinical decision support to improve performance on perioperative quality and process measures. Anesthesiol Clin 2011;29:57–69.
[43] Ehrenfeld JM, Wanderer JP, Terekhov M, et al. A perioperative systems design to improve intraoperative glucose monitoring is associated with a reduction in surgical site infections in a diabetic patient population. Anesthesiology 2017;126:431–40.

[44] Nair BG, Grunzweig K, Peterson GN, et al. Intraoperative blood glucose management: impact of a real-time decision support system on adherence to institutional protocol. J Clin Monit Comput 2016;30:301–12.
[45] Eden A, Pizov R, Toderis L, et al. The impact of an electronic reminder on the use of alarms after separation from cardiopulmonary bypass. Anesth Analg 2009;108:1203–8.
[46] Nair BG, Peterson GN, Newman SF, et al. Improving documentation of a beta-blocker quality measure through an anesthesia information management system and real-time notification of documentation errors. Jt Comm J Qual Patient Saf 2012;38(6):283–8.
[47] Nair BG, Peterson GN, Neradilek MB, et al. Reducing wastage of inhalation anesthetics using real-time decision support to notify of excessive fresh gas flow. Anesthesiology 2013;118(4):874–84.
[48] Kooij FO, Vos N, Siebenga P, et al. Automated reminders decrease postoperative nausea and vomiting incidence in a general surgical population. Br J Anaesth 2012;108:961–5.
[49] Nair BG, Newman SF, Peterson GN, et al. Feedback mechanisms including real-time electronic alerts to achieve near 100% timely prophylactic antibiotic administration in surgical cases. Anesth Analg 2010;111:1293–300.
[50] Sessler DI, Turan A, Stapelfeldt WH, et al. Triple-low alerts do not reduce mortality: a real-time randomized trial. Anesthesiology 2019;130:72–82.
[51] Wax DB, McCormick PJ, Joseph TT, et al. An automated critical event screening and notification system to facilitate preanesthesia record review. Anesth Analg 2018;126(2): 606–10.
[52] Sandberg WS, Sandberg EH, Seim AR, et al. Real-time checking of electronic anesthesia records for documentation errors and automatically text messaging clinicians improves quality of documentation. Anesth Analg 2008;106:192–201.
[53] Wax DB, McCormick PJ. A real-time decision support system for anesthesiologist end-of-shift relief. Anesth Analg 2017;124(2):599–602.
[54] Bhutiani M, Jablonski PM, Ehrenfeld JM, et al. Decision support tool improves real and perceived anesthesiology resident relief equity. Anesth Analg 2018;127(2):513–9.
[55] Nair BG, Newman SF, Peterson GN, et al. Smart Anesthesia Manager™ (SAM)–a real-time decision support system for anesthesia care during surgery. IEEE Trans Biomed Eng 2013;60(1):207–10.
[56] AlertWatch. Available at: http://www.alertwatch.com. Accessed April 24, 2019.
[57] Tremper KK, Mace JJ, Gombert JM, et al. Design of a novel multifunction decision support display for anesthesia care: AlertWatch® OR. BMC Anesthesiol 2018;18(1):16.
[58] Sathishkumar S, Lai M, Picton P, et al. Behavioral modification of intraoperative hyperglycemia management with a novel real-time audiovisual monitor. Anesthesiology 2015;123(1): 29–37.
[59] Klumpner TT, Kountanis JA, Langen ES, et al. Use of a novel electronic maternal surveillance system to generate automated alerts on the labor and delivery unit. BMC Anesthesiol 2018;18(1):78.
[60] Kheterpal S, Shanks A, Tremper KK. Impact of a novel multiparameter decision support system on intraoperative processes of care and postoperative outcomes. Anesthesiology 2018;128(2):272–82.
[61] Stol IS, Ehrenfeld JM, Epstein RH. Technology diffusion of anesthesia information management systems into academic anesthesia departments in the United States. Anesth Analg 2014;118:644–50.
[62] Dutton RP. Large databases in anaesthesiology. Curr Opin Anaesthesiol 2015;28: 697–702.
[63] Einav S, O'Connor M. Does only size matter or is there still a place for single-center studies in the era of Big Data? Anesth Analg 2016;123:1623–8.
[64] Simpao AF, Pruitt EY, Cook-Sather SD, et al. The reliability of manual reporting of clinical events in an anesthesia information management system (AIMS). J Clin Monit Comput 2012;26:437–9.

[65] Kool NP, van Waes JA, Bijker JB, et al. Artifacts in research data obtained from an anesthesia information and management system. Can J Anaesth 2012;59:833–41.
[66] Hoorweg AJ, Pasma W, van Wolfswinkel L, et al. Incidence of artifacts and deviating values in research data obtained from an anesthesia information management system in children. Anesthesiology 2018;128:293–304.
[67] Simpao AF, Ahumada LM, Gálvez JA, et al. A review of analytics and clinical informatics in health care. J Med Syst 2014;38:45.
[68] Wazir A, Shukla A, Dutton RP. Patient satisfaction in anesthesia: implementation, relevance, and identification of meaningful measures. Adv Anesth 2018;36(1):23–37.
[69] Levin MA. Building a perioperative data warehouse. Available at: https://www.stahq.org/userfiles/ckfiles/files/downloads/554/193/75/Levin_STA_periop_data_warehouse.pdf. Accessed April 26, 2019.
[70] Hofer IS, Gabel E, Pfeffer M, et al. A systematic approach to creation of a perioperative data warehouse. Anesth Analg 2016;122:1880–4.
[71] Colquhoun DA, Naik BI, Durieux ME, et al, MPOG Investigators. Management of 1-lung ventilation-variation and trends in clinical practice: a report from the multicenter perioperative outcomes group. Anesth Analg 2018;126(2):495–502.
[72] Nagrebetsky A, Dutton RP, Ehrenfeld JM, et al. Variation in frequency of intraoperative arterial, central venous and pulmonary artery catheter placement during kidney transplantation: an analysis of invasive monitoring trends. J Med Syst 2018;42:66.
[73] Lobaugh LMY, Martin LD, Schleelein LE, et al. Medication errors in pediatric anesthesia: a report from the wake up safe quality improvement initiative. Anesth Analg 2017;125(3): 936–42.
[74] Glover CD, Fernandez AM, Huang H, et al, Pediatric Craniofacial Collaborative Group. Perioperative outcomes and management in midface advancement surgery: a multicenter observational descriptive study from the Pediatric Craniofacial Collaborative Group. Paediatr Anaesth 2018;28(8):710–8.
[75] Burjek NE, Nishisaki A, Fiadjoe JE, et al, PeDI Collaborative Investigators. Videolaryngoscopy versus fiber-optic intubation through a supraglottic airway in children with a difficult airway: an analysis from the multicenter pediatric difficult intubation registry. Anesthesiology 2017;127(3):432–40.
[76] Dutton RP. Quality management and registries. Anesthesiol Clin 2014;32(2):577–86.
[77] Gálvez JA, Rothman BS, Doyle CA, et al. A narrative review of meaningful use and anesthesia information management systems. Anesth Analg 2015;121:693–706.
[78] Few S. Dashboard design: beyond meters, gauges and traffic lights. Business Intelligence Journal 2005;10:18–24.
[79] Kimball R, Ross M, Thornthwaite W, et al, editors. The data warehouse lifecycle toolkit. 2nd edition. Hoboken (NJ): Wiley; 2008.
[80] Wanderer JP, Gruss CL, Ehrenfeld JM. Using visual analytics to determine the utilization of preoperative anesthesia assessments. Appl Clin Inform 2015;6(4):629–37.
[81] Gálvez JA, Ahumada L, Simpao AF, et al. Visual analytical tool for evaluation of 10-year perioperative transfusion practice at a children's hospital. J Am Med Inform Assoc 2014;21(3):529–34.
[82] Simpao AF, Ahumada LM, Gálvez JA, et al. The timing and prevalence of intraoperative hypotension in infants undergoing laparoscopic pyloromyotomy at a tertiary pediatric hospital. Paediatr Anaesth 2017;27:66–76.
[83] Kang Y, Gorg C, Stasko J. How can visual analytics assist investigative analysis? Design implications from an evaluation. Visualization and Computer Graphics. IEEE Trans Vis Comput Graph 2011;17:570–83.
[84] Hofer IS, Halperin E, Cannesson M. Opening the black box: understanding the science behind big data and predictive analytics. Anesth Analg 2018;127(5):1139–43.

[85] Rahman QA, Janmohamed T, Pirbaglou M, et al. Defining and predicting pain volatility in users of the manage my pain app: analysis using data mining and machine learning methods. J Med Internet Res 2018;20(11):e12001.
[86] Fairley M, Scheinker D, Brandeau ML. Improving the efficiency of the operating room environment with an optimization and machine learning model. Health Care Manag Sci 2018. [Epub ahead of print].
[87] Kendale S, Kulkarni P, Rosenberg AD, et al. Supervised machine-learning predictive analytics for prediction of postinduction hypotension. Anesthesiology 2018;129(4):675–88.
[88] Sippl P, Ganslandt T, Prokosch HU, et al. Machine learning models of post-intubation hypoxia during general anesthesia. Stud Health Technol Inform 2017;243:212–6.
[89] Jalali A, Simpao AF, Gálvez JA, et al. Prediction of periventricular leukomalacia in neonates after cardiac surgery using machine learning algorithms. J Med Syst 2018;42(10):177.
[90] Gálvez JA, Jalali A, Ahumada L, et al. Neural network classifier for automatic detection of invasive versus noninvasive airway management technique based on respiratory monitoring parameters in a pediatric anesthesia. J Med Syst 2017;41(10):153.
[91] Lee CK, Hofer I, Gabel E, et al. Development and validation of a deep neural network model for prediction of postoperative in-hospital mortality. Anesthesiology 2018;129(4):649–62.
[92] Hatib F, Jian Z, Buddi S, et al. Machine-learning algorithm to predict hypotension based on high-fidelity arterial pressure waveform analysis. Anesthesiology 2018;129(4):663–74.
[93] Jelacic S, Bowdle A, Nair BG, et al. A system for anesthesia drug administration using barcode technology: the Codonics Safe Label System and Smart Anesthesia Manager. Anesth Analg 2015;121:410–21.
[94] Kim UR, Peterfreund RA, Lovich MA. Drug infusion systems: technologies, performance, and pitfalls. Anesth Analg 2017;124:1493–505.
[95] Klumpner TT, Bauer ME, Kheterpal S. Current applications of big data in obstetric anesthesiology. Curr Opin Anaesthesiol 2017;30:300–5.
[96] Liem VGB, Hoeks SE, van Lier F, et al. What we can learn from Big Data about factors influencing perioperative outcome. Curr Opin Anaesthesiol 2018;31(6):723–31.

Advances in Anesthesia 37 (2019) 163–186

ADVANCES IN ANESTHESIA

Spinal Cord and Peripheral Nerve Stimulation for Painful Disorders

William David Mauck, MD, Christine L. Hunt, DO, Oludare O. Olatoye, MD, Nafisseh S. Warner, MD, Tim J. Lamer, MD*

Department of Anesthesiology and Perioperative Medicine, Division of Pain Medicine, Mayo Clinic, 200 First Street Southwest, Rochester, MN 55905, USA

Keywords

- Spinal cord stimulation • Peripheral nerve stimulation
- Dorsal root ganglion stimulation • Neuromodulation

Key points

- Spinal cord stimulation is effective therapy for many intractable chronic pain conditions, including complex regional pain syndrome, failed back surgery syndrome, and peripheral neuropathy.
- Peripheral nerve stimulation is effective therapy for more localized chronic pain conditions, targeting specific nerves and/or more discrete anatomic structures.
- Stimulation technology is evolving at a rapid pace and, associated with the improvements in technology, outcomes are improving and indications are expanding.

INTRODUCTION: NATURE OF THE PROBLEM

Chronic pain represents one of the most significant public health problems in terms of the number of patients affected and in terms of health care costs. Pain affects more Americans than diabetes, heart disease, and cancer combined. Despite advances in treatments, a significant number of patients with chronic pain fail to improve with standard conservative medical therapy.

Disclosures: No extramural funding was used for any portion of this work. Dr T.J. Lamer serves on an advisory board for Vertos Medical and in the past, has participated in funded research with funding from Boston Scientific and Medtronic corporations. All funds were/are paid to his institution. The authors have no other conflicts.

*Corresponding author. *E-mail address:* lamer.tim@mayo.edu

https://doi.org/10.1016/j.aan.2019.08.010
0737-6146/19/

Medical therapy is the most common treatment of chronic pain, but a recent evidence-based review of medical therapy for chronic neuropathic pain concluded that, "Existing pharmacologic treatments for NP pain are limited, with no more than 40-60% of patients obtaining partial relief of their pain." [1] As many as half of all patients who present to their medical providers with common chronic painful conditions such as diabetic peripheral neuropathy, postherpetic neuralgia, complex regional pain syndrome (CRPS), and failed back surgery syndrome (FBSS) with a neuropathic component therefore fail to improve sufficiently with conservative pain care measures.

Neuromodulation is one of the fastest growing fields in medicine. Spinal cord stimulation (SCS) and peripheral nerve stimulation (PNS) are two common examples of neuromodulation used for the treatment of pain and have been shown to be effective treatment options for many patients with refractory neuropathic pain. However, studies indicate that most clinicians are not familiar with these treatment options [2–5]. As a result, many patients who could potentially benefit are not referred to a qualified pain specialist to determine candidacy for these therapies. Because many chronic pain conditions are lifelong problems, failure to refer patients for appropriate therapy potentially subjects them to needless long-term suffering. Another important consideration is that SCS and PNS may be viable and effective alternatives to oral opioid therapy for patients with intractable or complex pain problems. Opioid treatment of chronic pain is common and has contributed to the opioid crisis in the United States. The widespread use of opioids for chronic pain has occurred despite only limited evidence for long-term efficacy. In the past, SCS and PNS were considered by many physicians to be later-stage pain therapies, mainly because of the invasive nature of the therapy. More recently, because of the limited efficacy and the myriad problems associated with chronic opioid therapy, many pain specialists rightfully consider implementing SCS or PNS earlier in the treatment algorithm for patients with intractable pain [3,6]. The major advantage of these therapies is that medications are not involved and the side effects commonly associated with pain medications, such as drowsiness, mental clouding, and constipation, are avoided. This article discusses SCS and PNS therapies that have been shown to be effective treatments for patients with refractory chronic pain. It covers indications, contraindications, and technical details of the procedures, clinical outcomes, and adverse events.

INDICATIONS AND CONTRAINDICATIONS

Spinal cord stimulation

SCS is indicated for the treatment of chronic pain resulting from many common as well as uncommon conditions, including FBSS or postlaminectomy pain, CRPS, painful diabetic peripheral neuropathy, neuropathic pain of the trunk and/or limbs, chronic intractable back and lower limb pain, and refractory angina pectoris. Originally approved for the indication of neuropathic pain of the trunk and legs in 1989, indications for its use have grown as this therapeutic modality has become better understood and mechanisms of its delivery have evolved and improved (Table 1). Traditional or conventional (also referred

Table 1
Indications for spinal cord stimulation

Indication	Proposed neuromodulation modality
FBSS	SCS (conventional/HF)
CRPS	SCS (conventional/HF) or DRG[a]
PDN	SCS, consider DRG[a] for severe plantar foot pain
Neuropathic trunk or limb pain	SCS, consider DRG[a] for focal pain
LBP + lower limb pain	SCS (consider HF for primarily axial low back pain)
RAP	SCS (conventional/HF)

Abbreviations: DRG, dorsal root ganglion stimulation; HF, high frequency; LBP, low back pain; PDN, painful diabetic neuropathy; RAP, refractory angina pectoris.
[a] Note that DRG is approved for low thoracic and lumbar placement only.

to as tonic stimulation) SCS involves the delivery of an electric current (measured in milliamperes) to the dorsal columns in the form of perceptible paresthesia that is traditionally tailored to patient comfort by the adjustment of parameters including amplitude, pulse width, and frequency. This delivery is achieved by percutaneous or surgical placement of electrodes in the epidural space, with electrode contacts positioned either according to reported patient response (a process commonly referred to as paresthesia mapping) in the case of conventional SCS, or electrodes positioned over the T9 to T10 disc space in the case of high-frequency (HF) SCS. This process is discussed in greater detail later. Burst stimulation is another form of SCS involving alteration of the parameters listed earlier in the development of a proprietary and distinct waveform. Burst SCS has been shown in large-scale randomized controlled trials (RCTs) to be an effective therapy for back and/or limb pain. There is some preliminary evidence that the burst waveform may modulate the affective or medial pathway components of pain, including pain vigilance and awareness, possibly via activation of the dorsal anterior cingulate cortex [7].

Dorsal root ganglion (DRG) stimulation involves placement of lead contacts in the neural foramen from an epidural approach, and, because of this specific location in close proximity to the DRG, the amount of electricity that is delivered is much smaller (measured in microamperes). DRG stimulation is distinct from SCS, but both involve neuromodulation of spinal structures that can be achieved using a percutaneous approach, with some overlapping indications. Note that there are multiple emerging indications for DRG, including pelvic pain, visceral pain, postherniorrhaphy pain, and other focal pain syndromes. DRG stimulation is currently US Food and Drug Administration (FDA) approved only for lumbosacral placement (below T10).

From an anatomic standpoint, SCS may be the only viable option for advanced interventional therapies in cases in which spinal anatomy is altered to such a degree that further surgery is unlikely to improve the patient's symptoms or the patient's comorbidities are such that risks of further spine surgery outweigh potential benefits. Epidural access for lower limb or low back pain is typically at the thoracolumbar junction or L1 to L2 epidural space, often above the area of prior lumbar surgery. Epidural access for cervical pain is typically in the upper thoracic region and may be considered for patients with prior cervical surgery that has been accessed using an anterior approach as long as posterior elements, including the ligamentum flavum, remain intact. Anatomic considerations are discussed further later in the article.

As a neuromodulation therapy, SCS is most effective in treating pain with neuropathic or ischemic components. In general, it is most strongly indicated for medically refractory neuropathic pain of the trunk or limbs in patients with appropriate spinal anatomy for safe and effective lead placement.

Failed back surgery syndrome

FBSS is perhaps the most studied indication for SCS. Multiple prospective RCTs have shown the efficacy of FBSS, including superiority compared with reoperation as well as conventional medical management [8,9]. SCS may be effective not only in reducing pain following FBSS but also in improving anxiety, depression, and pain intensity, and reducing opioid usage [10]. Conventional paresthesia-based SCS as well as some of the newer stimulation paradigms, such as HF SCS and burst SCS, have all been shown to be effective therapies for FBSS [11].

Complex regional pain syndrome

Medically intractable CRPS is often debilitating and can create a challenging management problem. Presenting as a constellation of sudomotor, sensory, vasomotor, and trophic signs and symptoms caused by an inciting event (CRPS type II or causalgia) or without identifiable cause (CRPS type I), the mainstay of treatment includes physical therapy and activity modification, with refractory cases often requiring trials of various medications and injection therapies, including sympathetic nerve blocks that may achieve therapeutic efficacy. SCS is considered in refractory cases [12]. SCS has been shown to be effective in treating CRPS, including improvements in pain, quality of life, and satisfaction with SCS therapy [13]. DRG stimulation has also been shown to be effective in select patients with lower limb CRPS and superior to conventional SCS, provided pain symptoms follow an identifiable dermatomal pattern [14].

Diabetic peripheral neuropathy

SCS is also indicated for management of intractable painful diabetic neuropathy (PDN), improving pain as well as overall health and quality of life compared with conventional medical therapy [15]. SCS has been shown to be effective up to 5 years following implantation, particularly in cases in which the severity of PDN is not advanced [16]. Trials to date have investigated the use of conventional SCS for this indication, and inquiry into efficacy of HF versus conventional SCS is ongoing. Plantar foot pain may be difficult to capture with dorsal column SCS, and in such cases DRG stimulation may be considered for treatment of focal pain in PDN.

Low back pain

Although tonic stimulation historically has worked well for neuropathic limb pain, axial low back pain is often difficult to treat with conventional/tonic SCS. HF SCS has been shown to be effective for treatment of low back pain and superior in efficacy to tonic SCS for this indication [17]. The use of HF stimulation has introduced a highly effective therapy for many patients with axial low back pain with or without lower limb pain, and should be considered for patients with primarily low back pain who are otherwise appropriate candidates for neuromodulation provided there is not an anticipated need for repeated MRI.

Refractory angina pectoris

An FDA-approved indication for SCS, refractory angina pectoris (RAP) can be highly responsive to dorsal column SCS. Lead placement classically ranges from the lower cervical to upper thoracic region, and paresthesia mapping in tonic stimulation can be very helpful in confirming appropriate placement. SCS has been shown to be effective in improving angina symptoms, exercise duration, and nitrate consumption in patients with RAP [18–20]. As with all SCS indications, appropriate patient selection is critical. Implanting physicians considering SCS for treatment of RAP may find it beneficial to coordinate care with the patient's cardiologist in order to ensure appropriateness of therapy and that all diagnostic evaluation and medical treatment from a cardiovascular standpoint has been completed before consideration of trial and implantation. However, patients who have SCS placed for treatment of RAP should continue regular and appropriate cardiovascular follow-up. There is no evidence to suggest that SCS masks symptoms that are important in monitoring patients with angina symptoms.

Spinal cord stimulation: contraindications

A thorough evaluation including comprehensive history and physical examination is critical when considering patient candidacy for dorsal column SCS or DRG stimulation. From a diagnosis standpoint, neuromodulation is most effective for treatment of neuropathic or ischemic pain states, and patients with inflammatory disease or widespread myofascial pain are not as likely to experience a positive response to this therapy. MRI review should prioritize consideration of safety, and ensuring that the epidural space is adequate for safe lead placement may necessitate obtaining additional MRI of the thoracic spine in the case of treatment of lower limb or truncal pain. Intact posterior elements, including ligamentum flavum at the levels of access and final lead positioning, are necessary, and posterior spine surgery at these sites precludes percutaneous lead placement.

Beyond diagnostic and anatomic considerations, a psychological evaluation is recommended as a routine component of the comprehensive patient evaluation once a patient has been determined to be a potential candidate. Psychosocial factors such as untreated psychiatric disorders that may present barriers to successful treatment may be addressed through participation in psychotherapy, cognitive behavior therapy, or a comprehensive pain rehabilitation program. Conditions discovered during the course of psychological evaluation, such as severe psychiatric disorders or active addiction, should be addressed in the best interests of the patient, and appropriate referrals placed.

Medical comorbidities such as poorly controlled diabetes mellitus, an immunosuppressed state, poor cardiorespiratory health, or other health conditions that would pose a danger to the patient in terms of tolerance to anesthesia, positioning during trial and/or implantation, and healing during the postoperative period should be considered and appropriately managed. Trial should only proceed if any medical comorbidities can be adequately and safely addressed. Patients who are on anticoagulant or antiplatelet therapy or who otherwise have a bleeding diathesis must be able to have their anticoagulant or antiplatelet therapy held for the appropriate time period before and after trial and implant if it is safe to do so. Joint decision making with the patient's provider prescribing such medication is critical in considering this decision and whether it is safe from a medical standpoint to hold administration of this medication in the perioperative period.

When selecting SCS or DRG therapy, MRI compatibility is another important consideration. SCS devices are compatible to varying degrees, with some devices completely incompatible with MRI, such that the need for this imaging may necessitate explant of the entire device. The need for future MRI should be considered and discussed with the patient and may factor in to specific device selection. If a patient with an SCS system does need MRI, the patient needs to confirm with the implanting SCS physician that the SCS system has MRI compatibility. This confirmation involves knowing the SCS brand and model number as well as where the SCS leads and generators are implanted. All SCS devices have an MRI safety checklist from the manufacturer and, for those devices that have MRI compatibility, the devices have an MRI safe mode that in some cases involves having the device turned off. Again, this can be confirmed by discussing with the implanting SCS physician and/or the SCS company representatives.

Peripheral nerve stimulation

Indications

PNS involves percutaneous lead placement proximal to an identified peripheral nerve lesion. This therapy may be appropriate to consider in patients with pain of the trunk or limbs with an identified peripheral nerve target accessible percutaneously. Historically, standard SCS leads were placed peripherally to achieve PNS, but there are now devices available exclusively for PNS that are more securely anchored and specific to the indication of PNS. As such, PNS is again becoming more widely considered for the indication of intractable neuropathic pain involving peripheral nerves, cranial neuralgias, and CRPS [21]. Small-scale studies have suggested that some cases of axial pain with neuropathic features refractory to SCS may respond to subcutaneous PNS, but this has not been replicated in larger RCTs [22]. More recently, implantation of PNS devices targeting the medial branches of lumbar dorsal rami were reported in 9 patients who reported pain relief up to 4 months following implantation [23]. Poststroke hemiplegic shoulder pain is perhaps the most well-studied and classic indication for PNS, with patients showing improvement in pain and range of motion up to 2 years following implantation along the axillary nerve of the affected shoulder [24]. A variety of small-scale studies and reports have identified multiple potential targets for PNS, including postherniorrhaphy pain (including ilioinguinal and genitofemoral neuralgia) upper and lower limb peripheral nerve pain including CRPS, SI joint pain, as well as postoperative knee pain [25–30].

Contraindications

Considerations described earlier in terms of psychological factors, anticoagulation status, immunosuppressed state, and other medical comorbidities, including diabetes mellitus, must be considered as part of determining patient candidacy. PNS placement often does not require significant anesthesia beyond local infiltration, and patient positioning for implantation is highly variable depending on the target. As such, PNS is generally a safer procedure but medical contraindications must still be considered based on the target for device placement.

THERAPEUTIC OPTIONS AND SURGICAL TECHNIQUES

Spinal cord stimulation

SCS modalities can be differentiated based on the type of electrical charge delivered to surrounding tissues, the frequency (in Hertz) at which this charge is delivered, the presence or perception of paresthesia, and stimulation target of the implanted device. The 3 major types of SCS are:

- Conventional paresthesia-based SCS
- High-frequency 10 (HF10) SCS
- DRG stimulation

The hardware components of all SCS systems include an electrode array or lead, an implantable pulse generator (IPG), and a portable wireless programmer (Fig. 1). Most pulse generators are implanted generators similar to a pacemaker battery, but some SCS systems use an external generator that communicates with the stimulator leads via radiofrequency (RF) energy or Bluetooth. Before implantation, the ideal candidate undergoes a trial period usually between 5 and 7 days. For the trial, temporary percutaneous SCS leads are inserted into the epidural space with the IPG remaining external to the skin with sterile dressing, and during the trial period the patient is instructed to perform usual/typical daily activities to determine the pain-relieving impact of the temporary stimulation. The purpose of this trial is to determine whether the patient obtains sufficient clinical improvement to justify a surgical implantation. At the completion of the trial, the temporary leads are removed and a decision is made about whether or not the pain improvement was sufficient

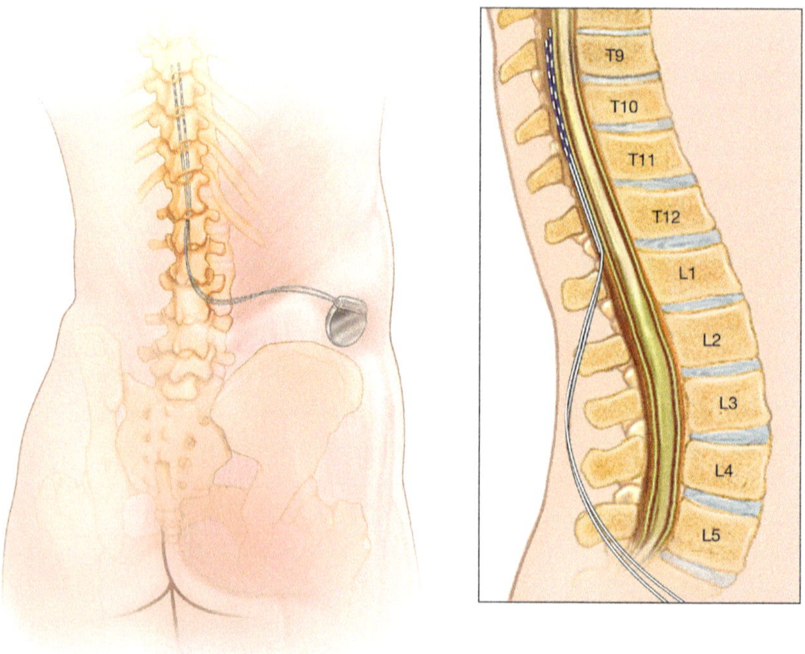

Fig. 1. Components of a typical spinal cord stimulator system. There are 2 spinal cord stimulator leads in the epidural space and an implanted pulse generator in the right lower flank/upper buttock area. (Used with permission of Mayo Foundation for Medical Education and Research. All rights reserved.)

to move forward with the surgically inserted permanent system. The period between the trial phase and implantation phase is typically 3 to 4 weeks.

Conventional spinal cord stimulation

Conventional SCS, often referred to as tonic SCS, is a modality that uses stimulation frequencies between 40 and 200 Hz. This modality is most commonly thought to function through the gate control mechanism [31]. It involves stimulation of large dorsal column sensory fibers, specifically A-beta fibers, which in turn suppresses both central hyperexcitability and the activation of pain signaling from A-delta and C fibers. There is also evidence that SCS increases the levels of several dorsal horn neurotransmitters that are known to be pain modulating, including serotonin, norepinephrine, GABA (gamma-aminobutyric acid), and acetylcholine. SCS has been shown to modulate sensitized dorsal horn wide-dynamic-range neurons, which are implicated in many neuropathic pain states. SCS may also antidromically stimulate the peripheral release of vasodilatory neurotransmitters, including CGRP (calcitonin gene-related peptide) and nitric oxide [32]. Action potentials generated by stimulation subsequently lead to the generation of paresthesia over the area of pain.

Conventional SCS percutaneous technique usually involves placement of 2 SCS leads into the dorsal epidural space following epidural access using a Touhy needle under fluoroscopy guidance (Fig. 2A). The patency of the epidural space is verified via advanced imaging, such as a computed tomography or MRI scan obtained preprocedurally. The target level and laterality bias of the placed leads depend on the location of the patient's symptoms. The leads are advanced under fluoroscopy guidance via anteroposterior view to the target level. To ensure the leads are maintained in the dorsal epidural space, lateral and contralateral oblique views are used. The appropriate physiologic location of the epidural leads is verified by ensuring the presence of paresthesia over the area of pain, a process known as paresthesia mapping [33]. In addition to the percutaneous SCS lead placement technique described earlier, an alternative is an open surgical technique to place leads directly into the epidural space via a laminotomy/laminectomy. There are pros and cons to each technique. The percutaneous technique is less invasive, whereas the open surgical approaches can be useful for patients with challenging spine anatomy.

High-frequency spinal cord stimulation

HF10 SCS is another modality of SCS that involves the use of a proprietary waveform with frequency at 10,000 Hz [34]. Stimulation at this higher frequency does not generate the perception of paresthesia. The exact mechanism of action of this stimulation mode remains to be elucidated. Possible targets in the pain perception pathway include modulation of wide-dynamic-range neurons, regulation of inhibitory and excitatory neurotransmitter release from the dorsal horn, and activation of the inhibitory descending pathway [32,35].

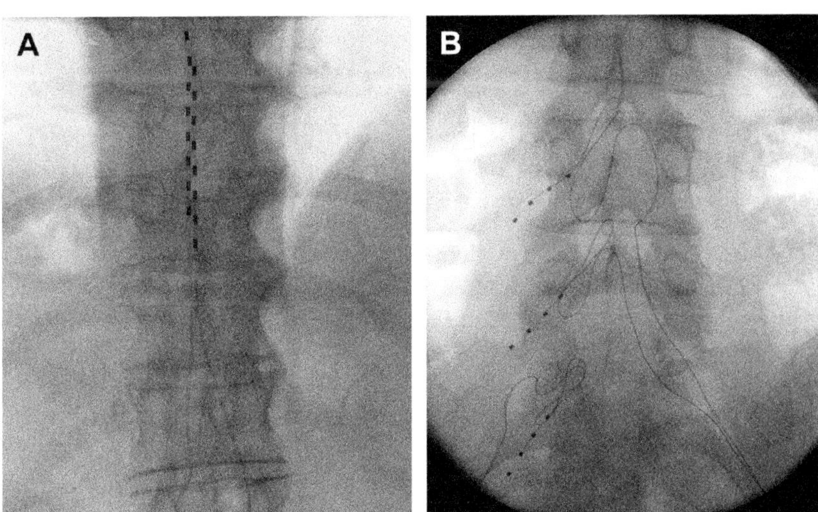

Fig. 2. (*A*) Radiograph of 2 epidural spinal cord stimulator leads. (*B*) Radiograph of 3 DRG stimulator leads placed at L4 (forth lumbar level), L5, and S1 on the left side.

In terms of technique, the placement of HF10 SCS leads into the dorsal epidural space is similar to that of conventional SCS described earlier. However, unlike conventional SCS, physiologic or paresthesia mapping over the area of pain is not needed or required following lead placement with the HF10 system. The leads are usually placed in the anatomic midline with electrodes staggered to facilitate optimal coverage. Impedance level, which is a surrogate of resistance and energy requirement in the system, is usually confirmed along with radiographic evidence.

When percutaneous devices are placed, minimal procedural analgesia is usually needed during placement of conventional and HF10 leads for both trials and implantation. Subcutaneous infiltration of the epidural needle access area with local anesthetic only usually suffices for SCS trials and can be supplemented with other intravenous agents (conscious sedation vs monitored anesthesia care) as deemed appropriate by the anesthetic provider. Regardless of the anesthetic modality used, the patient needs to be awake and interactive during SCS lead maneuvering in the epidural space to ensure that the patient is able to communicate any signs of neural integrity violation to the proceduralist. If a laminotomy/laminectomy procedure is performed for lead placement, then general anesthesia is most commonly used, and intraoperative neurophysiologic monitoring is used.

Dorsal root ganglion stimulation

Despite the well-established benefits of conventional and HF10 SCS in the treatment of neuropathic pain associated with FBSS and CRPS, adequate coverage of focal and localized areas of pain, such as in the feet, inguinal area, and groin, can be challenging [36]. Targeting the DRG that supplies these specific locations has been proposed as an effective alternative [37]. The DRG is usually located in or close to the neural foramen. It contains cell bodies of primary sensory neurons and regulates the transmission of sensory signals from the periphery via primary afferent nerves to the dorsal spinal cord column, acting essentially as a gatekeeper [38]. DRG stimulation has been shown to decrease neuronal hyperexcitability and chronic neuropathic pain signaling [39].

Similar to dorsal column SCS, the ideal patient for DRG stimulation undergoes a trial period before implantation of the IPG. However, major differences exist between DRG stimulation and dorsal column SCS. DRG leads have 4 electrode contacts, unlike those used in dorsal column systems, which vary in the number of electrode contacts (8–16 electrodes). Because of the close lead proximity to the DRG needed for stimulation, as well as small foraminal opening, DRG lead placement can be stimulating and uncomfortable in awake patients. As such, the procedure can be safely performed under general anesthesia with the use of neurophysiologic monitoring in the form of evoked potentials such as electromyography, motor evoked potentials, and somatosensory evoked potentials [40].

For DRG lead placement, the target DRG is identified based on the patient's pain location [41]. For example, foot pain is typically treated with L5 and

S1 DRG lead placement, and inguinal pain is treated with T12 and/or L1 lead placement. Skin entry with the epidural needle is performed on the contralateral side of the target DRG, usually about 2 vertebral levels caudal in the upper lumbar area (L1–L4). For the L5 DRG, skin entry is performed 1 vertebral level down on the contralateral side. Entry into the sacral DRG is performed ipsilateral at the same level [34]. Once the lead is in its final position in the dorsal neural foramen, strain relief loops (S loops) are made in a cephalocaudal fashion to anchor the leads and prevent migration (Fig. 2B). As with dorsal column SCS, optimal placement of DRG leads is confirmed via stimulation, level of impedance, and radiographic imaging. Similar to HF10 SCS, DRG stimulation is usually paresthesia free.

Peripheral nerve stimulation

Neuromodulation targeting peripheral nerves has been used to treat painful conditions for decades [42]. Although SCS and DRG target regional pain conditions, PNS allows the targeting of specific nerves and thus more discrete anatomic structures and painful conditions.

Historically, PNS required an open surgical procedure with direct visualization of the nerve to place a flat plate electrode either next to or around the nerve [43]. It then required the lead be tunneled to a location where the IPG could be connected and surgically implanted under the skin. In 1999, Weiner and Reed [44] published a case series showing that cylindrical SCS leads placed percutaneously could successfully treat occipital neuralgia. Ultrasonography-guided placement of a cylindrical lead PNS system was first reported by Huntoon and Burgher [45] in 2009, thus visualizing the nerve and lead juxtaposed without an open procedure. However, specific systems designed specifically for PNS did not exist. Instead, SCS systems were used, which still required a lead tunneled to distant location, typically the abdomen, trunk, buttock, or thigh, where a surgical pocket housed a large IPG. These systems were prone to lead migration, skin erosion, and surgical revision or explant [46].

Only recently have specifically designed systems for percutaneous PNS become widely available. Design-specific PNS systems are less invasive, easier to place, and may be less intrusive for patients. As interest in innovative PNS systems grows, so has the interest in applying it to patients with postamputation pain, shoulder pain, knee pain, postherniorrhaphy pain, and low back pain [23,24,29,47–51].

Although these systems are uniquely different from one another, they have at least 2 common components: a lead and an external energy source. The leads are typically placed with ultrasonography guidance next to the nerve of interest. The leads vary in their diameter, number of contacts, three-dimensional structure, and whether they activate via monopolar or bipolar stimulation. They all have a unique, nonsurgically deployable anchoring system not found in the SCS systems historically used. This feature reduces the risk of lead migration but still keeps the procedure minimally invasive. They have also eliminated the IPG and replaced it with an external pulse transmitter (EPT) or external stimulator. Amplitude, pulse width, and frequency can all be adjusted to varying degrees but with much fewer waveform choices compared with SCS. Each of these devices has a patient-controlled handheld remote that can adjust the amplitude, power the device on/off, and in some cases cycle pre-set programs.

StimRouter (Bioness, Inc., Valencia, CA) and StimQ PNS (Stimwave, Inc., Pompano Beach, FL) are two design-specific PNS systems that use a fully implanted lead and an EPT system. The distal end of the lead with the electrodes is placed percutaneously via ultrasonography guidance near the nerve. The proximal end of the lead is then brought near the skin surface while remaining fully implanted under the skin. This proximal end acts as a receiver for the EPT, which uses wireless power transfer and RF signals to power and communicate with the implanted lead.

The StimRouter implant procedure requires only a 1.0-cm incision placed approximately 7 to 10 cm from the nerve of interest. The 15-cm lead containing 3 electrodes is introduced through this incision and often by ultrasonography guidance to the proper location near the identified nerve. Proximity to the nerve is confirmed with electrical stimulation. Once confirmed, the proximal end of the lead is tunneled subcutaneously from the incision site approximately 5 cm away. The EPT can then be placed on the skin over the proximal end of the tunneled lead, which contains the receiver. This EPT is secured by means of a disposable electrode pad with a skin adhesive.

The StimQ PNS lead has the potential advantage of 4 electrodes and uses a wearable antenna assembly that is approximated over the implanted lead receiver by means of an adjustable belt, band, or fabric.

SPRINT PNS System (SPR Therapeutics, Inc., Cleveland, OH) is a temporary PNS system with an externalized lead and pulse generator. It is intended for 60 days of use, at which point the entire lead is removed and therapy ceases. The lead is a 0.- mm diameter, open-coiled design with a single monopolar contact. The coiled structure is designed to encourage fibrotic ingrowth, minimizing migration. No incision is required. Instead an introducer and stimulating probe are inserted simultaneously through the skin to the target nerve. Once nerve proximity is confirmed with electrical stimulation, the stimulating probe is removed and replaced with the lead. In addition, the introducer is removed over the externalized lead. The lead is then trimmed to a manageable length, connected to the external pulse generator, and secured with an occlusive bandage. The bandage is changed every 2 to 3 days until the lead is removed.

Each of these specifically designed PNS systems is potentially less invasive, requires less energy, and is more cost-effective than central nervous system stimulation or using an SCS-adapted system for PNS. However, there still may be a role for an SCS-adapted system when multiple leads are desired or an external power source is not tolerated.

CLINICAL OUTCOMES

Spinal cord stimulation outcomes

Several RCTs and systematic reviews have shown the effectiveness of SCS in chronic pain states (Table 2). In a prospective RCT with 2-year follow-up, SCS combined with physical therapy provided superior pain improvement compared with physical therapy alone in patients with refractory CRPS [52]. SCS was superior to repeat lumbar spine surgery in patients who had recurrent or persistent pain after previous lumbar spine surgery [8]. Forty-seven percent of patients randomized to SCS versus 12% randomized to repeat surgery achieved greater than 50% pain improvement. In an RCT of 100 patients with intractable neuropathic pain in the setting of failed lumbar spine surgery, Kumar and colleagues [9] showed that SCS plus medical therapy was superior to medical therapy alone. In this trial, 45% of patients with SCS compared with only 5% of medical management patients achieved greater than 50% relief of pain at 1-year follow-up. The patients with SCS also experienced significant improvements in function and quality of life compared with the medical therapy group. A recently completed RCT comparing 2 different types of SCS for patients with chronic back and leg pain showed that both types of SCS offered significant improvement in pain and function. HF SCS (using a stimulation frequency of 10,000 Hz) was superior to conventional, low-frequency stimulation, with 65% of patients in the HF group experiencing significant pain relief at 18-month follow-up, a result that was statistically superior to conventional low-frequency SCS [17]. Several recent trials, including 2 RCTs, have shown SCS to be effective for the treatment of intractable pain related to PDN [15,53]. Each of the chronic pain conditions discussed earlier is notoriously difficult and stubborn to manage effectively with medical therapy. Patients that do not respond to reasonable attempts at conservative medical therapy should be referred sooner rather than later for consideration of neuromodulation approaches. As further evidence of efficacy, recent systematic review and meta-analysis of RCTs showed that SCS was significantly more likely than medical therapy to relieve pain in a variety of chronic painful conditions, including PDN, CRPS, and intractable spine and limb pain.

In addition to the common chronic neuropathic pain problems described earlier, SCS has been shown to provide significant pain reduction in patients with other challenging painful medical conditions; for example, painful vasospastic diseases [54,55]. Patients with refractory chest pain from coronary vasospasm or small vessel disease that is not amenable to definitive coronary stenting or bypass procedures can have significant improvement in pain and quality of life, and reduced physician and emergency room visits following treatment with SCS [18–20]. SCS has shown promise in several other difficult-to-treat chronic neuropathic pain states, including postherpetic neuralgia, postamputation pain, and limb pain secondary to peripheral vascular disease.

A recently published prospective randomized multicenter trial comparing traditional SCS with DRG spinal stimulation in patients with CRPS showed

and randomized to either the treatment group (N = 45) with stimulation on or the control group (N = 49) with stimulation off. At 3 months, 38% of the treatment group and 10% of the control group achieved greater than 30% pain relief (P<.0048). At crossover the treatment group again showed significant pain relief. The treatment group also experienced significant improvement in quality of life and satisfaction at 3 months.

In a feasibility case series, Rauck and colleagues [60] treated chronic postamputation pain, both phantom and residual limb pain, with an externalized PNS system. Nine patients completed a 2-week stimulation trial with a 4-week follow-up. Greater than 30% pain relief was achieved for 8 of the 9 patients at 2 weeks and 7 patients at 4 weeks. The mean worst daily postamputation pain was reduced 56% at 2 weeks (P>.005) and at 4 weeks (P>.005). Prospective postamputation studies are forthcoming.

The first report to use ultrasonography-guided PNS for acute postoperative pain has recently been described. Five patients with refractory post–total knee arthroplasty (TKA) pain (≤60 days postoperative) were treated with the SPRINT PNS system for less than 1 hour. Four of the 5 patients had immediate and complete pain relief. One patient had immediate 67% pain reduction. No further follow-up was reported [49]. This study was followed by a second case series of 5 patients with similar inclusion criteria and treatment parameters. Immediate and significant pain relief (≥50%) at rest was reported in 4 of the 5 patients [48]. A third case series describes placing SPRINT PNS leads in 7 patients before undergoing a TKA. Continuous stimulation was initiated within 20 hours of surgery for up to 6 weeks postsurgery. During the first postoperative week the average daily pain overall, at rest, and with ambulation was reported as mild (less than or equal to 4 out of 10) in 6 of 7 patients. Pain remained mild at weeks 2, 3, and 4 in 6 of 7 patients. Four of the 7 patients discontinued opioids within the first week compared with recent studies reporting that more than 80% of patients continue to take opioids 2 weeks after a TKA. Functional recovery was assessed using the 6-minute walk test (6MWT). Within 2 weeks from surgery, 6 of 7 subjects were able to perform the 6MWT at a level equal (≥95% baseline performance) to their preoperative performance, and by 12 weeks all subjects were at baseline [50].

Recent studies report PNS stimulation for varied causes of chronic shoulder pain. In a case series for hemiplegic shoulder pain, 28 patients were trialed for 3 weeks with an externalized PNS system placed to stimulate the axillary nerve motor points. Sixteen patients had a successful trial (≥2-point pain reduction). Ten of these had no return of baseline pain within 6 months. Five eventually advanced to have an IPG placed for long-term PNS stimulation. At 6 and 12 months, all 5 participants experienced at least 50% pain reduction and, at 24 months, 4 experienced at least 50% pain reduction. The implant group also experienced significant improvement in pain interference at 6, 12, and 24 months [24]. Another cohort of patients with subacromial impingement syndrome was trialed for 3 weeks with an externalized PNS system. Pain, disability, shoulder range of motion, and pain interference improved significantly through the 16-week follow-up [47].

A recent case series reported that 6 of 9 patients with chronic low back pain achieved clinically significant reduction ($\geq$50%) in average pain intensity at 4 weeks while using the SPRINT PNS system. Four months after the start of treatment, 4 of 5 experienced clinically significant reduction in average and worst pain intensity. The Oswestry Disability Index was significantly reduced ($\geq$10 points) in 67% patients at 4 weeks, and 60% of patients at 4 months [23].

COMPLICATIONS AND ADVERSE EVENTS

Although generally considered safe procedures that are typically performed in an outpatient setting, placement of implantable SCS and PNS devices is associated with multiple potential complications, as described in Table 3. Complications may be biological or mechanical [46]. In addition, they may be shared by both types of devices or be specific to SCS or PNS. Major biological complications, similar to many invasive pain procedures, include infection, bleeding, and nerve injury, with the most common biological complication being infection, estimated to occur in approximately 2.5% to 10% of SCS placements and up to 6% of PNS placements [15,53,61–63]. Lead complications are the most common mechanical complications, and include lead migration, fracture, and failure. Lead migrations, likely the most common lead complication, may require reprograming or surgical revision. Distinct from lead complications, there are also complications related to the device itself, including malfunction or early battery failure. Moreover, complications may occur at the time of device placement, including injury to vasculature, nerves, or other nearby structures, or months to even years later. Additional concerns include device intolerability, new or worsening pain after device placement (including over the generator site), lack of improvement in physical function despite appropriate device placement, and issues related to insurance coverage. Although characterization of these potential complications (eg, incidence, typical severity) remains largely incomplete, patients must be counseled on these before implantation and consent must be explicitly documented.

SUMMARY AND FUTURE CONSIDERATIONS

The future of spinal cord and peripheral nerve stimulation therapies

The past 25 years have seen remarkable advancements in advanced interventional pain-relieving devices such as PNS and SCS. Outcomes are improving because of improvements in equipment, generator software, and surgical techniques. For example, approximately 50% of patients improved with SCS in the early RCTs for SCS (older hardware and software platforms), whereas more recent trials with improved technology such as HF10 SCS, burst SCS, and DRG stimulation, have shown success in 75% to 80% of patients [14,17,75]. There has been a rapid expansion of therapies, with many new devices approved in the last few years, including HF SCS, DRG stimulation, and minimally invasive PNS devices. There are several promising therapies

Table 3
Potential complications and adverse events from spinal cord stimulation and peripheral nerve stimulation

Category	Shared complications	SCS-specific complications	PNS-specific complications
Biological	Infection	Infection (2.5%–10%) [15,53,61,62]	Infection (1%–6%) [63–66]
	Superficial surgical site	Meningitis	
	Deep surgical site		
	Bleeding	Bleeding	Bleeding
	Major (eg, neurologic deficit, requires surgery)	Neuraxial hematoma ($\leq$0.3%) [67,68]	
	Minor (eg, superficial hematoma)		
	Nerve injury	Nerve injury	Nerve injury
	Transient neuropraxia	Spinal cord injury	Peripheral nerve injury
	Permanent injury	Paralysis (0.03%) [67]	
	Miscellaneous	Miscellaneous	Miscellaneous
	Seroma	Erosion (0.2%) [67]	
	Allergic reactions		
	Fistula formation		
	Erosion		
Mechanical	Lead complications	Lead complications	Lead complications
	Migration	Migration (13%–23%) [62,67,69–71]	Migration
	Fracture	Fracture (6%–9%) [62,72,74]	Fracture (2% for ONS) [66]
	Failure		
	Device complications	Device complications	Device complications
	Malfunction		
	Early battery failure ($\leq$1.7%) [67]		
	Overstimulation		

Other	New pain Implant, lead anchor sites Neuropathic	New pain Implant, lead anchor sites (1%–12%) [15,54,62,67,72,73]	New pain Implant, lead sites (6% ONS) [66]
	Placement complications Injury to surrounding structures Vascular injury	Placement complications Dural puncture (0%–0.3%) [62,67] Nerve root or cord injury	Placement complications Peripheral nerve injury
	Additional concerns Device Intolerability Worsened pain after placement Lack of improvement in function Early removal (secondary to above) Lack of insurance coverage	—	—

Abbreviation: ONS, Occipital Nerve Stimulation.

in development [76]. One promising new technology currently in clinical trials in the United States and Australia involves an evoked compound action potential controlled closed-loop SCS system. This system uses real-time measurement of spinal cord neuronal stimulation to control the amount of SCS energy being delivered [76]. This technique allows more precise control of the dose or amount of electrical energy being delivered and has the potential for improved pain control and reduced generator/battery use (prolonged generator life).

Summary

Approximately 40 million people in the United States have chronic pain. Of these, approximately 10 million have what has been termed high-impact chronic pain, meaning pain that has lasted 3 months or longer and is accompanied by at least 1 major activity restriction, such as being unable to work outside the home, go to school, or do household chores [77]. Most of these patients are treated with medications as the mainstay of therapy, but most medically treated patients continue to report ongoing pain. In addition to suboptimal pain relief, many patients experience significant adverse events from medications, including drowsiness, cognitive decline, and constipation. SCS and PNS therapy are well-established techniques that have been used for more than 25 years, and many RCTs and systematic reviews have shown superiority of these techniques compared with medical therapy for many common chronic pain conditions. Patients with intractable pain that have failed reasonable attempts at conservative pain care measures should be referred to a qualified interventional pain specialist to determine candidacy for the procedures discussed in this article.

References

[1] Dworkin RH, O'Connor AB, Backonja M, et al. Pharmacologic management of neuropathic pain: evidence-based recommendations. Pain 2007;132:237–51.
[2] Compton AK, Shah B, Hayek SM. Spinal cord stimulation: a review. Curr Pain Headache Rep 2012;16:35–42.
[3] Deer TR. Spinal cord and peripheral nerve stimulation should be used earlier in the treatment algorithm for neuropathic pain. Pain Manag 2011;1:7–10.
[4] Kumar K, Abbas M, Rizvi S. The use of spinal cord stimulation in pain management. Pain Manag 2012;2:125–34.
[5] Kumar K, Rizvi S. Cost-effectiveness of spinal cord stimulation therapy in management of chronic pain. Pain Med 2013;14:1631–49.
[6] Deer TR. Neurostimulation should be used as a method of reducing or eliminating opioids in the treatment of chronic pain: the digital drug revolution. Expert Rev Med Devices 2013;10: 697–9.
[7] De Ridder D, Plazier M, Kamerling N, et al. Burst spinal cord stimulation for limb and back pain. World Neurosurg 2013;80(5):642–9.
[8] North RB, Kidd DH, Farrokhi F, et al. Spinal cord stimulation versus repeated lumbosacral spine surgery for chronic pain: a randomized, controlled trial. Neurosurgery 2005;56(1):98–106.
[9] Kumar K, Taylor RS, Jacques L, et al. Spinal cord stimulation versus conventional medical management for neuropathic pain: a multicentre randomised controlled trial in patients with failed back surgery syndrome. Pain 2007;132(1–2):179–88.

[10] Robb LP, Cooney JM, McCrory CR. Evaluation of spinal cord stimulation on the symptoms of anxiety and depression and pain intensity in patients with failed back surgery syndrome. Ir J Med Sci 2017;186(3):767–71.
[11] De Andres J, Monsalve-Dolz V, Fabregat-Cid G, et al. Prospective, randomized blind effect-on-outcome study of conventional vs high-frequency spinal cord stimulation in patients with pain and disability due to failed back surgery syndrome. Pain Med 2017;18(12): 2401–21.
[12] Poree L, Krames E, Pope J, et al. Spinal cord stimulation as treatment for complex regional pain syndrome should be considered earlier than last resort therapy. Neuromodulation 2013;16(2):125–41.
[13] Visnjevac O, Costandi S, Patel BA, et al. A comprehensive outcome-specific review of the use of spinal cord stimulation for complex regional pain syndrome. Pain Pract 2017;17(4):533–45.
[14] Deer TR, Levy RM, Kramer J, et al. Dorsal root ganglion stimulation yielded higher treatment success rate for complex regional pain syndrome and causalgia at 3 and 12 months: a randomized comparative trial. Pain 2017;158(4):669–81.
[15] de Vos CC, Meier K, Zaalberg PB, et al. Spinal cord stimulation in patients with painful diabetic neuropathy: a multicentre randomized clinical trial. Pain 2014;155(11):2426–31.
[16] van Beek M, Geurts JW, Slangen R, et al. Severity of neuropathy is associated with long-term spinal cord stimulation outcome in painful diabetic peripheral neuropathy: five-year follow-up of a prospective two-center clinical trial. Diabetes Care 2018;41(1):32–8.
[17] Kapural L, Yu C, Doust MW, et al. Novel 10-kHz high-frequency therapy (HF10 Therapy) is superior to traditional low-frequency spinal cord stimulation for the treatment of chronic back and leg pain: the SENZA-RCT randomized controlled trial. Anesthesiology 2015;123(4): 851–60.
[18] Imran TF, Malapero R, Qavi AH, et al. Efficacy of spinal cord stimulation as an adjunct therapy for chronic refractory angina pectoris. Int J Cardiol 2017;227:535–42.
[19] Pan X, Bao H, Si Y, et al. Spinal cord stimulation for refractory angina pectoris: a systematic review and meta-analysis. Clin J Pain 2017;33(6):543–51.
[20] Eldabe S, Thomson S, Duarte R, et al. The effectiveness and cost-effectiveness of spinal cord stimulation for refractory Angina (RASCAL Study): a pilot randomized controlled trial. Neuromodulation 2016;19(1):60–70.
[21] Nayak R, Banik RK. Current innovations in peripheral nerve stimulation. Pain Res Treat 2018;2018:9091216.
[22] Burgher AH, Huntoon MA, Turley TW, et al. Subcutaneous peripheral nerve stimulation with inter-lead stimulation for axial neck and low back pain: case series and review of the literature. Neuromodulation 2012;15(2):100–6 [discussion 6-7].
[23] Gilmore CA, Kapural L, McGee MJ, et al. Percutaneous Peripheral Nerve Stimulation (PNS) for the treatment of chronic low back pain provides sustained relief. Neuromodulation 2019;22(5):615–20.
[24] Wilson RD, Bennett ME, Nguyen VQC, et al. Fully implantable peripheral nerve stimulation for hemiplegic shoulder pain: a multi-site case series with two-year follow-up. Neuromodulation 2018;21(3):290–5.
[25] Shaw A, Sharma M, Zibly Z, et al. Sandwich technique, peripheral nerve stimulation, peripheral field stimulation and hybrid stimulation for inguinal region and genital pain. Br J Neurosurg 2016;30(6):631–6.
[26] Bouche B, Manfiotto M, Rigoard P, et al. Peripheral nerve stimulation of brachial plexus nerve roots and supra-scapular nerve for chronic refractory neuropathic pain of the upper limb. Neuromodulation 2017;20(7):684–9.
[27] Dewandre Q, Dubuisson A, Kaschten B, et al. Refractory neuropathic pain from a median nerve injury: spinal cord or peripheral nerve stimulation? A case report. Acta Neurol Belg 2019. [Epub ahead of print].

[28] Guentchev M, Preuss C, Rink R, et al. Long-term reduction of sacroiliac joint pain with peripheral nerve stimulation. Oper Neurosurg (Hagerstown) 2017;13(5):634–9.
[29] Ilfeld BM, Gilmore CA, Grant SA, et al. Ultrasound-guided percutaneous peripheral nerve stimulation for analgesia following total knee arthroplasty: a prospective feasibility study. J Orthop Surg Res 2017;12(1):4.
[30] Ilfeld BM, Said ET, Finneran JJT, et al. Ultrasound-guided percutaneous peripheral nerve stimulation: neuromodulation of the femoral nerve for postoperative analgesia following ambulatory anterior cruciate ligament reconstruction: a proof of concept study. Neuromodulation 2019;22(5):621–9.
[31] Melzack R, Wall PD. Pain mechanisms: a new theory. Science 1965;150:971–9.
[32] Lamer TJ, Deer TR, Hayek SM. Advanced Innovations for Pain. Mayo Clin Proc 2016;91: 246–58.
[33] Verrills P, Sinclair C, Barnard A, et al. A review of spinal cord stimulation systems for chronic pain. J Pain Res 2016;9:481–92.
[34] Russo M, Van Buyten JP. 10-kHz high-frequency SCS therapy: a clinical summary. Pain Med 2015;16(5):934–42.
[35] Linderoth B. Spinal cord stimulation: a brief update on mechanisms of action. Eur J Pain Suppl 2009;3(2):89–93.
[36] Abejon D, Feler C. Is impedance a parameter to be taken into account in spinal cord stimulation? Pain Physician 2007;10:533–40.
[37] Morgalla M, Fortunato M, Lepski G, et al. Dorsal Root Ganglion Stimulation (DRGS) for the treatment of chronic neuropathic pain: a single-center study with long-term prospective results in 62 cases. Pain Physician 2018;21(4):E377–87.
[38] Pope JE, Deer TR, Kramer J. A systematic review: current and future directions of dorsal root ganglion therapeutics to treat chronic pain. Pain Med 2013;14:1477–96.
[39] Krames ES. The dorsal root ganglion in chronic pain and as a target for neuromodulation: a review. Neuromodulation 2015;18:24–32.
[40] Falowski S, Dianna A. Neuromonitoring protocol for spinal cord stimulator cases with case descriptions. Int J Acad Med 2016;2:132–44.
[41] Vancamp T, Levy RM, Pena I, et al. Relevant anatomy, morphology, and implantation techniques of the dorsal root ganglia at the lumbar levels. Neuromodulation 2017;20: 690–702.
[42] Wall PD, Swert WH. Temporary abolition of pain in man. Science 1967;155(3758): 108–9.
[43] Nashold B, Goldner J, Mullen J, et al. Long-term pain control by direct peripheral nerve stimulation. J Bone Joint Surg Am 1982;64:1–10.
[44] Weiner R, Reed K. Peripheral neurostimulation for control of intractable occipital neuralgia. Neuromodulation 1999;2:217–21.
[45] Huntoon M, Burgher A. Ultrasound-guided permanent implantation of peripheral nerve stimulation (PNS) system for neuropathic pain of the extremities: original cases and outcomes. Pain Med 2009;10:1369–77.
[46] Eldabe S, Buchser E, Duarte R. Complications of spinal cord stimulation and peripheral nerve stimulation techniques: a review of the literature. Pain Med 2016;17(2):325–36.
[47] Wilson R, Harris M, Gunzler D, et al. Percutaneous peripheral nerve stimulation for chronic pain in subacromial impingement syndrome: a case series. Neuromodulation 2014;17: 771–6.
[48] Ilfeld B, Grant S, Gilmore C, et al. Neurostimulation for postsurgical analgesia: a novel system enabling ultrasound-guided percutaneous peripheral nerve stimulation. Pain Pract 2017;17(7):892–901.
[49] Ilfeld B, Ball S, Gabriel R, et al. A feasibility study of percutaneous peripheral nerve stimulation for the treatment of postoperative pain following total knee arthroplasty. Neuromodulation 2019;22(5):653–60.

[50] Ilfeld B, Ball S, Cohen S, et al. Percutaneous peripheral nerve stimulation to control postoperative pain, decrease opioid use, and accelerate functional recovery following orthopedic trauma. Mil Med 2019;184:157–64.
[51] Elahi F, Reddy C, Ho D. Ultrasound guided peripheral nerve stimulation implant for management of intractable pain after inguinal herniorrhaphy. Pain Physician 2015;18:E31–8.
[52] Kemler MA, De Vet HC, Barendse GA, et al. The effect of spinal cord stimulation in patients with chronic reflex sympathetic dystrophy: two years' follow-up of the randomized controlled trial. Ann Neurol 2004;55:13–8.
[53] Slangen R, Schaper NC, Faber CG, et al. Spinal cord stimulation and pain relief in painful diabetic peripheral neuropathy: a prospective two-center randomized controlled trial. Diabetes Care 2014;37:3016–24.
[54] Ubbink DT, Vermeulen H. Spinal cord stimulation for non-reconstructable chronic critical leg ischaemia. Cochrane Database Syst Rev 2013;(2):CD004001.
[55] Deogaonkar M, Zibly Z, Slavin KV. Spinal cord stimulation for the treatment of vascular pathology. Neurosurg Clin N Am 2014;25:25–31.
[56] Kemler MA, Raphael JH, Bentley A, et al. The cost-effectiveness of spinal cord stimulation for complex regional pain syndrome. Value Health 2010;13:735–42.
[57] Kumar K, Rizvi S, Nguyen R, et al. Impact of wait times on spinal cord stimulation therapy outcomes. Pain Pract 2014;14:709–20.
[58] Rizvi S, Kumar K. Spinal cord stimulation for chronic pain: the importance of early referral. Pain Manag 2014;4:329–31.
[59] Deer T, Pope J, Benyamin R, et al. Prospective, multicenter, randomized, double-blinded, partial crossover study to assess the safety and efficacy of the novel neuromodulation system in the treatment of patients with chronic pain of peripheral nerve origin. Neuromodulation 2016;19:91–100.
[60] Rauck R, Cohen S, Gilmore C, et al. Treatment of post-amputation pain with peripheral nerve stimulation. Neuromodulation 2014;17:188–97.
[61] Hoelzer BC, Bendel MA, Deer TR, et al. Spinal cord stimulator implant infection rates and risk factors: a multicenter retrospective study. Neuromodulation 2017;20:558–62.
[62] Kumar K, Hunter G, Demeria D. Spinal cord stimulation in treatment of chronic benign pain: challenges in treatment planning and present status, a 22-year experience. Neurosurgery 2006;58:481–96 [discussion: 96].
[63] Paemeleire K, Van Buyten JP, Van Buynder M, et al. Phenotype of patients responsive to occipital nerve stimulation for refractory head pain. Cephalalgia 2010;30:662–73.
[64] Sator-Katzenschlager S, Fiala K, Kress HG, et al. Subcutaneous target stimulation (STS) in chronic noncancer pain: a nationwide retrospective study. Pain Pract 2010;10:279–86.
[65] Verrills P, Vivian D, Mitchell B, et al. Peripheral nerve field stimulation for chronic pain: 100 cases and review of the literature. Pain Med 2011;12:1395–405.
[66] Saper JR, Dodick DW, Silberstein SD, et al. Occipital nerve stimulation for the treatment of intractable chronic migraine headache: ONSTIM feasibility study. Cephalalgia 2011;31:271–85.
[67] Cameron T. Safety and efficacy of spinal cord stimulation for the treatment of chronic pain: a 20-year literature review. J Neurosurg 2004;100:254–67.
[68] Moeschler SM, Warner NS, Lamer TJ, et al. Bleeding complications in patients undergoing percutaneous spinal cord stimulator trials and implantations. Pain Med 2016;17:2076–81.
[69] North RB, Recinos VR, Attenello FJ, et al. Prevention of percutaneous spinal cord stimulation electrode migration: a 15-year experience. Neuromodulation 2014;17:670–6 [discussion: 6–7].
[70] Taylor RS, Van Buyten JP, Buchser E. Spinal cord stimulation for chronic back and leg pain and failed back surgery syndrome: a systematic review and analysis of prognostic factors. Spine (Phila Pa 1976) 2005;30:152–60.

[71] Taylor RS, Van Buyten JP, Buchser E. Spinal cord stimulation for complex regional pain syndrome: a systematic review of the clinical and cost-effectiveness literature and assessment of prognostic factors. Eur J Pain 2006;10:91–101.
[72] Mekhail NA, Mathews M, Nageeb F, et al. Retrospective review of 707 cases of spinal cord stimulation: indications and complications. Pain Pract 2011;11:148–53.
[73] Turner JA, Loeser JD, Deyo RA, et al. Spinal cord stimulation for patients with failed back surgery syndrome or complex regional pain syndrome: a systematic review of effectiveness and complications. Pain 2004;108:137–47.
[74] Kumar K, Taylor RS, Jacques L, et al. The effects of spinal cord stimulation in neuropathic pain are sustained: a 24-month follow-up of the prospective randomized controlled multicenter trial of the effectiveness of spinal cord stimulation. Neurosurgery 2008;63:762–70 [discussion: 770].
[75] Deer T, Slavin KV, Amirdelfan K, et al. Success using neuromodulation with BURST (SUNBURST) study: results from a prospective, randomized controlled trial using a novel burst waveform. Neuromodulation 2018;21:56–66.
[76] Maheshwari A, Pope JE, Deer TR, et al. Advanced methods of spinal stimulation in the treatment of chronic pain: pulse trains, waveforms, frequencies, targets, and feedback loops. Expert Rev Med Devices 2019;16:95–106.
[77] Pitcher MH, Von Korff M, Bushnell MC, et al. Prevalence and profile of high-impact chronic pain in the United States. J Pain 2018;20:146–60.

Advances in Anesthesia 37 (2019) 187–205

ADVANCES IN ANESTHESIA

Ultrasound-Guided Fascial Plane Blocks of the Thorax

Pectoral I and II, Serratus Anterior Plane, and Erector Spinae Plane Blocks

Ki Jinn Chin, MMed, FRCPC[a,*], Amit Pawa, FRCA, EDRA[b], Mauricio Forero, MD, FIPP[c], Sanjib Adhikary, MD[d]

[a]Department of Anesthesia, Toronto Western Hospital, University of Toronto, 399 Bathurst Street, McL 2-405, Toronto, Ontario M5T 2S8, Canada; [b]Anaesthetic Department, Guy's & St Thomas' NHS Foundation Trust, St Thomas' Hospital, Westminster Bridge Road, London SE1 7EH, UK; [c]Department of Anesthesia, Faculty of Health Sciences, McMaster University, 1280 Main Street West, Hamilton, Ontario L8S 4L8, Canada; [d]Department of Anesthesiology and Perioperative Medicine, Penn State College of Medicine, 500 University Drive, Hershey, PA 17033, USA

Keywords

• Thoracic wall • Chest wall • Ultrasound • Regional anesthesia • Nerve blocks • Pectoral • Serratus anterior • Erector spinae

Key points

- Ultrasound-guided thoracic fascial plane blocks provide alternative analgesic options to well-established techniques such as thoracic epidural and paravertebral blocks.
- These techniques are relatively simple and safe to perform and thus can increase the use of regional anesthesia by less-experienced practitioners and in turn extend the benefits of regional anesthesia to more patients.
- Fascial plane blocks rely on indirect and passive spread of injected local anesthetic to nerves located either within the fascial plane itself or within adjacent compartments; variable efficacy is therefore expected.
- The evidence base for these techniques is accumulating steadily and initial results are very encouraging, especially for added benefit compared with systemic analgesia alone.

Continued

Disclosure Statement: Dr A. Pawa consults for B Braun Medical Ltd & Metaphor and has received honoraria from GE Healthcare. The other authors have nothing to disclose.

*Corresponding author. *E-mail address:* gasgenie@gmail.com

https://doi.org/10.1016/j.aan.2019.08.007

Continued

- These techniques involve injection of relatively large volumes of local anesthetic into well-vascularized areas, and practitioners must be vigilant for delayed local anesthetic systemic toxicity from systemic absorption.

INTRODUCTION

Regional analgesia of the thorax has traditionally been limited to thoracic epidural analgesia, thoracic paravertebral blocks, or intercostal blocks. In recent years, a new class of ultrasound-guided peripheral nerve blocks has emerged. Instead of targeting individual nerves or plexi, local anesthetic is injected into a plane between 2 fascial layers and subsequently spreads to nerves traveling within that interfascial plane or to adjacent tissue compartments containing nerves. At the time of this writing, the most prevalent of these fascial plane blocks of the thorax are the pectoral type I and II blocks (PECS I and II), serratus anterior plane (SAP) block, and the erector spinae plane (ESP) block. The aim of this article is to describe the technical performance of each block and summarize the indications, current evidence base, and future avenues for research.

ANATOMIC CONSIDERATIONS

The innervation of the thorax is primarily derived from the T1-T6 spinal nerves. These divide soon after emerging from the intervertebral foramina into dorsal rami, which ascend posteriorly to innervate the muscles and skin (that lie along the vertebral column) of the back, and ventral rami, which are continuous with the intercostal nerves (Fig. 1). Each intercostal nerve travels anteriorly in the intercostal space between internal and innermost intercostal muscles and along the inner and caudal aspect of the relevant rib. Numerous branches arise along the course of each intercostal nerve to supply the various bony and muscular structures of the thoracic cage [1]. A lateral cutaneous branch arises from the main nerve trunk near the costal angle and close to the midaxillary line, ascends superficially through the overlying muscle layers to split into anterior and posterior divisions, and supplies the skin and subcutaneous tissues over the anterolateral and posterolateral thorax. The lateral cutaneous branch of the T2 spinal nerve is particularly important, as it is the main contributor to the intercostobrachial nerve, which innervates most of the axilla [2,3]. At the same time, it must be noted that there is significant communication and anastomosis between adjacent spinal nerves and their branches, and thus the pattern of sensory innervation to any given area of tissue is complex and nonsegmental. Each intercostal nerve terminates in an anterior cutaneous branch that innervates the parasternal area and midline, with a significant degree of crossover innervation [4].

Several other important nerves supply the thorax and may need to be targeted for complete analgesia or anesthesia [3]. The lower branches of the

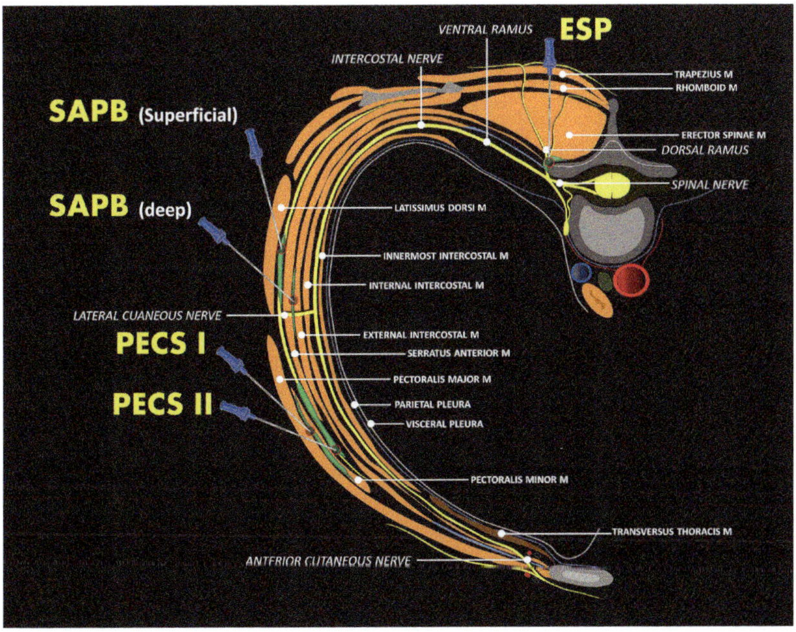

Fig. 1. Each thoracic spinal nerve divides into a dorsal ramus and ventral ramus. The dorsal ramus divides into medial, intermediate, and lateral branches as it ascends and supplies the posterolateral aspect of the thorax. The ventral ramus is continuous with the intercostal nerve and runs anteriorly between internal and innermost intercostal muscles. Numerous branches are given off along its course to supply muscles and rib. A lateral cutaneous branch arises at the costal angle in the midaxillary line and its anterior and posterior divisions innervate the anterolateral aspect of the superficial thoracic wall. The intercostal nerve terminates in the parasternal area as an anterior cutaneous branch. What is not illustrated are the numerous anastomoses between adjacent intercostal nerves and the crossover innervation that overlaps the midline. The location of injection of the PECS I and II blocks, the SAP block, and ESP block are illustrated. (*Courtesy of* Dr Vicente Roqués, Murcia, Spain.)

superficial cervical plexus, the supraclavicular nerves, provide cutaneous innervation of the "cape" of the shoulder and thus the anterior-superior aspect of the thorax. Several branches of the brachial plexus are responsible for motor and nociceptive innervation of thoracic muscles and are often overlooked as contributors to thoracic pain; these include (1) the medial and lateral pectoral nerves to pectoralis minor and major muscles, (2) the thoracodorsal nerve to latissimus dorsi, and (3) the long thoracic nerve to serratus anterior muscle.

ULTRASOUND-GUIDED PERIPHERAL NERVE BLOCK TECHNIQUES

General considerations

Ultrasound-guided peripheral nerve blocks of the thorax are, almost without exception, fascial plane blocks. As the individual nerves are too small to consistently visualize and target, the general principle is to inject relatively large volumes of local anesthetic (20–40 mL in adults; 0.2–0.4 mL/kg in children) into an interfascial plane, whereupon it spreads to nerves traveling within that plane or spreads to adjacent compartments (eg, the paravertebral space) that contain the target nerves. The pattern and extent of spread, not surprisingly, exhibits interindividual variability, which in turn contributes to a variable mass of local anesthetic reaching and acting on the nerves. As a result, differential blockade is a commonly observed phenomenon (analgesia > sensory > motor block) [5,6], and a degree of interindividual variation in block efficacy can be expected.

A common error with all fascial plane blocks is injection into muscle rather than the fascial plane. Intramuscular injection can be recognized by localized and diffused expansion of the muscular layer, as opposed to the appearance of an anechoic "pocket" of fluid that peels the muscle away from the adjacent bony or muscular layer. It is helpful to use nonactive fluid (normal saline or 5% dextrose) for *"hydrolocation"* of the correct plane, thus minimizing inaccurate deposition and "wastage" of local anesthetic.

Depending on the technique chosen, the point of injection may be in the anterior, lateral, or posterior thorax (see Fig. 1). The choice between techniques is therefore influenced not only by the desired neural targets but also by procedural considerations related to patient positioning, presence of wound dressings or drains, and interference with the surgical field.

Preparation for performance of any of these techniques must include informed consent, monitoring of vital signs (electrocardiogram, pulse oximetry, and noninvasive blood pressure), supplemental oxygen, intravenous access, and availability of emergency equipment including a local anesthetic systemic toxicity (LAST) rescue kit [7]. The blocks may be performed in awake, sedated, or anesthetized patients as the situation dictates.

Local anesthetic dosing

The efficacy of fascial plane blocks depends on physical spread, and thus local anesthetic volumes of 20 to 40 mL or 0.2 to 0.4 mL/kg are used for single-injection techniques. There is a potential risk of LAST from systemic absorption, and maximum recommended weight-based local anesthetic dose limits must be strictly observed. Epinephrine 5 mcg/mL should be routinely incorporated into the solution, even with ropivacaine. Epinephrine has been demonstrated to decrease the systemic absorption of local anesthetic when used for truncal blocks of the abdomen [8]. As these are primarily analgesic blocks, a dilute concentration (eg, 0.125%–0.25% bupivacaine or 0.2%–0.5% ropivacaine) is appropriate, with the exact concentration determined by the planned injectate volume and maximum allowable mass of drug.

If a continuous catheter technique is used, a loading dose of 20 mL or 0.2 mL/kg may be followed by either a continuous infusion regimen of dilute local anesthetic (0.125% bupivacaine or 0.2% ropivacaine) at 8 to 12 mL/h or a programmed intermittent bolus regimen of 10 to 15 mL every 1 to 3 hours.

PECTORAL I AND II BLOCKS

The PECS I block is an interpectoral injection of local anesthetic targeting medial and lateral pectoral nerves [9] (Box 1, Fig. 2). The PECS II block is a combination of interpectoral (ie, a PECS I) and subpectoral injections that additionally target lateral cutaneous branches of intercostal nerves, long thoracic nerves, and thoracodorsal nerves [9].

Positioning and approach

The patient should be in a supine position with the ipsilateral arm abducted 45 to 90 degrees. The head of the bed may be elevated for patient comfort and the

Box 1: PECS I and PECS II block performance

Preparation

- Consent
- Intravenous access
- Monitoring
- Sedation as required (if performing before GA)

Positioning

- Supine
- Arm abducted 45 to 90 degrees
- Head turned to contralateral side
- Ultrasound machine placed within line of sight

Approach

- High-frequency linear-array transducer
- 50 to 80 mm 22G block needle
- In-plane (superior medial to inferior lateral)

Technique Steps—PECS I—Interpectoral injection

- Place transducer in parasagittal plane below clavicle
- Identify PM and Pm, AA and AV, second to third ribs, and pleura below
- Rotate caudad part of transducer toward axilla over third and fourth ribs
- Deposit 10 to 20 mL or 0.1 to 0.2 mL/kg of LA between PM and Pm near pectoral branch of TAA

Technique Steps—PECS II—Subpectoral injection

- A PECS II block consists of the PECS I plus this subpectoral injection
- Advance needle from PECS I endpoint, through Pm to identify plane between Pm and SA
- Deposit 20 to 30 mL or 0.2 to 0.3 mL/kg of LA in this plane

Clinical Pearls

- Use color flow Doppler to identify blood vessels and aspirate before injection to avoid intravascular injection
- Identify the pleura before needle insertion
- Inject nonactive fluid (saline or dextrose) to identify fascial plane before LA injection so as to minimize wastage
- Use the rib as a landmark and backstop for safety when performing the subpectoral injection

Potential Complications

- Pneumothorax
- Vascular injury and hematoma formation
- LAST

Abbreviations: AA, axillary artery; AV, axillary vein; GA, general anesthesia; LA, local anesthetic; PM, pectoralis major; Pm, pectoralis minor; SA, serratus anterior; TAA, thoracoacromial artery.

patient's head turned to the contralateral side to aid needle insertion. The practitioner stands either at the head of the patient or on the contralateral side, ensuring that the ultrasound screen is appropriately positioned in the line of sight. A high-frequency linear-array transducer, 50 to 80 mm block needle,

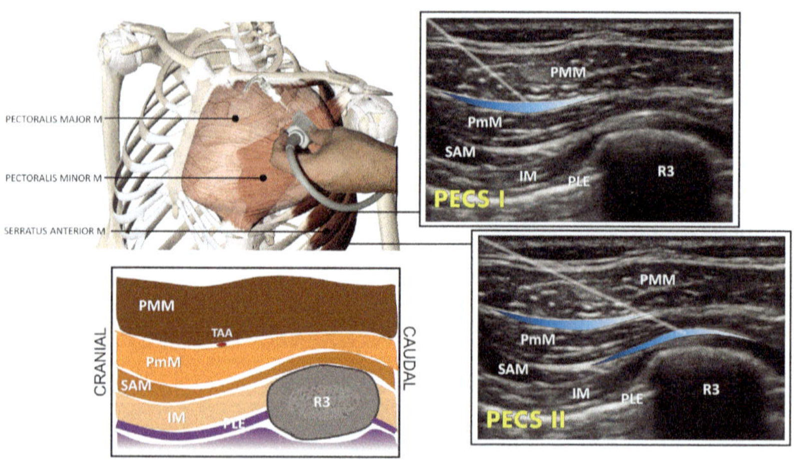

Fig. 2. When performing PECS I and II blocks, the transducer is placed in an oblique orientation parallel to the deltopectoral groove over the third rib (R3). In the PECS I block, the needle is advanced in-plane and an interpectoral injection is made between the pectoralis major muscle (PMM) and pectoralis minor muscle (PmM). In the PECS II block, the needle is advanced deeper, and a second additional injection is made between the PmM and serratus anterior muscle (SAM). The SAM is usually quite thin at this location and can be difficult to distinguish from the intercostal muscle (IM). Using the rib as a backstop prevents inadvertent puncture of the pleura (PLE). (*Courtesy of* Dr Vicente Roqués, Murcia, Spain.)

and in-plane needle approach technique in the superior-medial to inferior-lateral direction are recommended.

Technical steps

To perform the PECS I block, place the transducer in a midclavicular parasagittal plane and identify pectoralis major, minor, axillary vessels, and the pleura. Slide the transducer caudad to identify the second and third ribs and then rotate the inferior end of the transducer toward the axilla to bring it parallel to the deltopectoral groove. This rotation, combined with an in-plane needle approach, provides for better spread, particularly to the intercostobrachial nerve [9]. The needle tip is placed into the interpectoral fascial plane (between the pectoralis major and pectoralis minor) adjacent to the pectoral branch of the thoracoacromial artery and 10 to 20 mL or 0.1 to 0.2 mL/kg of local anesthetic is injected here (the higher volume is recommended if performing an isolated PECS I block).

To perform the PECS II block, in addition to the step discussed earlier, the needle is then advanced from its position in the interpectoral plane, through pec minor, into the fascial plane between pectoralis minor and serratus anterior; 20 to 30 mL or 0.2 to 0.3 mL/kg of local anesthetic is injected here. An alternative approach is to perform the deeper subpectoral injection first and then withdraw the needle into the interpectoral plane after this step.

Clinical pearls

- Use color flow Doppler to identify blood vessels in the path of the needle trajectory (cephalic vein and thoracoacromial artery) and aspirate before injection to avoid intravascular injection.
- Ensure identification of pleura before needle insertion
- Use the rib as a landmark and backstop for safety when performing the subpectoral injection.

Potential complications

- Pneumothorax
- Vascular injury to pectoral branch of thoracoacromial vessel or cephalic vein
- Local anesthetic systemic toxicity
- Temporary "winging" of the scapula if the long thoracic nerve is anesthetized (with subsequent motor block of the serratus anterior muscle) by local anesthetic spread

SERRATUS ANTERIOR PLANE BLOCK

The SAP block is an injection of local anesthetic into a fascial plane that is either superficial or deep to the serratus anterior muscle and primarily targets the lateral cutaneous and muscular branches of the intercostal nerves [10] (Box 2, Fig. 3). The long thoracic and thoracodorsal nerves lie in the fascial plane superficial to the serratus anterior muscle and can also be anesthetized. The superficial SAP block is anatomically similar to

Box 2: Serratus anterior plane block performance

Preparation

- Consent
- Intravenous access
- Monitoring
- Sedation as required (if performing before GA)

Positioning

- (1)Supine, arm abducted 90 degrees, or
- (2) Lateral, operative side up, arm flexed forward
- Ultrasound machine placed within line of sight

Approach

- High-frequency linear-array transducer
- 50 to 80 mm 22G block needle
- In-plane (cranial-to-caudal or caudal-to-cranial)

Technique Steps

- Place transducer in parasagittal plane below clavicle
- Identify the fourth rib by counting down
- Slide transducer laterally into the mid- or posterior axillary line over fourth rib
- Identify LD superficial to SA and SA superficial to the ribs and intercostal muscles
- Deposit 20 to 40 mL or 0.2 to 0.4 mL/kg of LA into either (1) the plane between LD and SA (superficial SAP block) or (2) the plane between SA and ribs (deep SAP block)

Clinical Pearls

- Larger LA volumes (30–40 mL) increase extent of blockade but also risk of LAST
- Inject nonactive fluid (saline or dextrose) to identify fascial plane before LA injection so as to minimize wastage
- Use the rib as a landmark and backstop for safety when performing the deep SAP block

Potential Complications

- Pneumothorax
- Vascular injury and hematoma formation
- LAST

Abbreviations: AA, axillary artery; AV, axillary vein; GA, general anesthesia; LA, local anesthetic; LD, latissimus dorsi; SA, serratus anterior; SAP, serratus anterior plane.

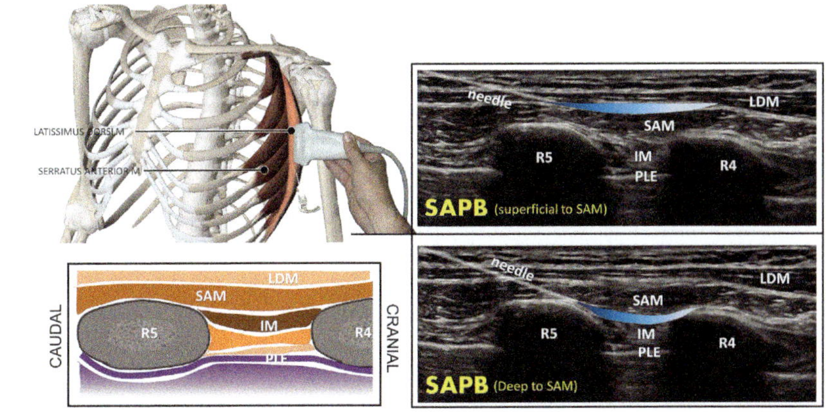

Fig. 3. When performing the SAP block, the probe is placed in a parasagittal plane over the fourth and fifth ribs (R4 and R5) in the midaxillary or posterior axillary line. In the superficial SAP block, the needle is advanced in-plane in either a caudal-to-cranial direction (illustrated here) or a cranial-to-caudal direction and an injection is made between the latissimus dorsi muscle (LDM) and the serratus anterior muscle (SAM). In the deep SAP block, the needle is advanced through SAM and an injection is made between SAM and the intercostal muscle (IM) and ribs. Note that the SAM at this level is thicker and more visible than in the PECS II block. The rib should be used as a backstop to prevent inadvertent puncture of the pleura (PLE). (*Courtesy of* Dr Vicente Roqués, Murcia, Spain.)

the subpectoral injection in the PECS II block. There is currently little evidence to support the superiority of the superficial over deep SAP block or vice versa [11,12], although it may be more intuitive to perform the deep SAP block if analgesia of the deeper bony and muscular structures is desired. Local anesthetic may also be deposited into both superficial and deep planes if desired.

Positioning and approach

The SAP block may be performed anywhere in the anatomic area between the anterior and posterior axillary line and the second to seventh ribs. The patient may be placed in either (1) a supine position with the ipsilateral arm abducted 90 degrees or (2) a lateral decubitus position with the operative side uppermost and the ipsilateral arm flexed forward out of the way. The practitioner stands either at the head of the patient or on one side, ensuring that the ultrasound screen is appropriately positioned in the line of sight. A high-frequency linear-array transducer, 50 to 80 mm block needle, and an in-plane needle approach in either a cranial-to-caudal or a caudal-to-cranial direction (a choice based primarily on ergonomics) are recommended.

Technical steps

The SAP block is generally performed at the level of the fourth rib; this can be identified by placing the transducer in a parasagittal plane just inferior to the clavicle and counting down from the second rib. The probe is moved laterally into the midaxillary or posterior axillary line, and the serratus anterior muscle is identified as the muscular layer overlying the anechoic rib shadow. Latissimus dorsi lies superficial to the serratus anterior muscle and will be thicker and more evident in the posterior axillary line. The needle tip is placed into the fascial plane either superficial or deep to the serratus anterior muscle, and 20 to 40 mL of local anesthetic is injected.

Clinical pearls

- Larger injectate volumes increase the extent of blockade [13,14] but also increase the risk of LAST.
- When performing a deep SAP block, it is advisable to aim for contact with the rib so as to minimize the risk of inadvertent pleural puncture
- If performing injection into both superficial and deep planes, injection into the deep plane first is recommended because superficial injection can hinder subsequent visualization of deeper structures.

Potential complications

- Pneumothorax
- Vascular injury to thoracodorsal artery that lies in the plane superficial to serratus anterior
- Local anesthetic systemic toxicity
- Temporary "winging" of the scapula if the long thoracic nerve is anesthetized by local anesthetic spread

ERECTOR SPINAE PLANE BLOCK

The ESP block is an injection of local anesthetic into the fascial plane between the erector spinae muscle and the tips of the transverse processes (Box 3, Fig. 4). The dorsal rami of spinal nerves pass through this plane and are effectively anesthetized. Blockade of the ventral rami and their branches is achieved by local anesthetic spread anteriorly into the paravertebral and epidural space [15–17]; there may also be lateral spread to the posterior divisions of the lateral cutaneous branches [18]. The targeted vertebral level should be congruent with the center of the desired area of coverage; however, a single-injection spreads to anesthetize at least 3 and as many as 6 to 8 spinal nerve territories [15,16], and thus targeting the T4 or T5 level is appropriate in most cases.

Positioning and approach

The ESP block may be performed in a lateral, sitting, or prone position as access to the patient's back is required. A high-frequency linear-array or lower-frequency curved-array transducer may be used; the choice is determined by depth from skin to transverse processes. This is usually 4 cm or less in adults at the midthoracic region (T4–T6) but is greater at higher levels (T1–T3), and thus a curved-array transducer may occasionally be required for optimal image quality. An in-plane needle parasagittal approach in either a cranial-to-caudal or a caudal-to-cranial direction (a choice based primarily on ergonomics) is recommended.

Box 3: Erector spinae plane block performance

Preparation
- Consent
- Intravenous access
- Monitoring
- Sedation as required (if performing before GA)

Positioning
- (1) Lateral decubitus (both sides accessible from the same position), or
- (2) Sitting, or
- (3) Prone
- Ultrasound machine placed within line of sight

Approach
- High-frequency linear-array transducer
- 50 to 80 mm 22G block needle
- In-plane (cranial-to-caudal or caudal-to-cranial)

Technique Steps
- Identify target vertebral level (usually T4 or T5) by counting down from C7 spinous process or scanning down from first rib
- Place transducer in parasagittal plane 2 to 3 cm lateral to spinous processes
- Identify TPs by their squared-off profile and absence of clearly visible pleural line between them
- Insert the needle in a shallow trajectory (30–40°) to contact the far edge of the target TP
- Deposit 20 to 30 mL or 0.2 to 0.3 mL/kg of LA into the plane between ESM and TPs.

Clinical Pearls
- Transverse view of vertebrae can aid identification of the tip of the TP
- Shift the needle, and not the transducer, to achieve needle-beam alignment without losing visualization of the target TPs
- Inject nonactive fluid (saline or dextrose) to identify fascial plane before LA injection so as to minimize wastage
- Advance the needle slightly deeper off the edge of the TP if necessary, to achieve accurate fluid deposition in the plane

Potential Complications
- Pneumothorax
- LAST

Abbreviations: AA, axillary artery; AV, axillary vein; ESM, erector spinae muscle; GA, general anesthesia; LA, local anesthetic; TP, transverse process.

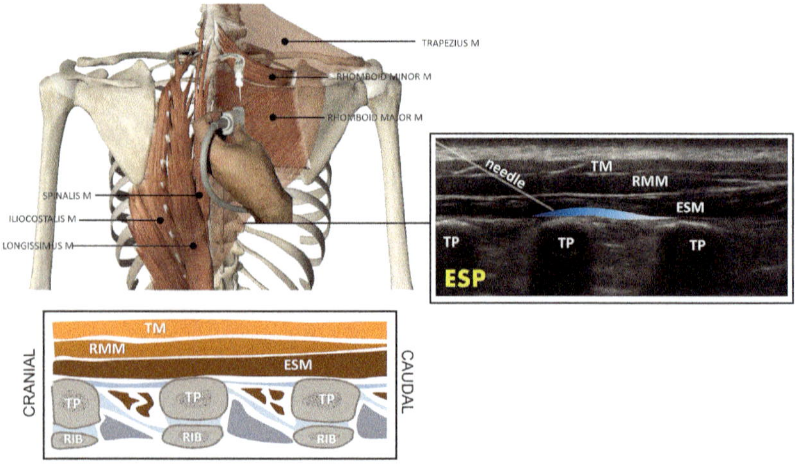

Fig. 4. When performing the ESP block, the probe is placed in a parasagittal plane over the tips of the transverse processes (TP). These are distinguished from the ribs by a more squared-off profile and absence of a hyperechoic pleural line between them. The needle is advanced in-plane in either a cranial-to-caudal direction (illustrated here) or a caudal-to-cranial direction through the trapezius muscle (TM), rhomboid major muscle (RMM), and erector spinae muscle (ESM), and an injection is made between the ESM and the TPs. The TP can be used as a back-stop to prevent excessively deep insertion, but occasionally the needle tip may have to be advanced slightly deeper off the edge of the TP to enter the fascial plane and produce the characteristic linear spread pattern of injectate. (*Courtesy of* Dr Vicente Roqués, Murcia, Spain.)

Technical steps

The desired target vertebral level is identified by either palpation of the C7 spinous process or ultrasonographic visualization of the first rib and counting down from there. The transducer is placed on the patient's back in a parasagittal plane 2 to 3 cm lateral to the midline spinous processes. The transverse processes are distinguished from the proximal ribs by their profile, which is squared-off rather than rounded, and the absence of a clearly visible pleural line between adjacent transverse processes. In the event of uncertainty, the probe can be placed initially in a transverse plane to visualize the contours of spinous process, lamina, and transverse process. The location of the transverse process tip is then marked on the skin before transducer rotation into the parasagittal plane. The fascial plane between the deep surface of erector spinae muscle and the posterior surface of the transverse processes is identified.

The needle tip is advanced in a shallow trajectory (30–40°) to contact the lateral edge of the target transverse process and placed into the fascial plane deep to erector spinae muscle; 20 to 30 mL or 0.2 to 0.3 mL/kg of local anesthetic is injected here.

Clinical pearls

- A rule of thumb for identifying the T6 transverse process is that rhomboid major muscle tapers off into its inferior border at this level.

- In-plane needle-beam alignment should not involve shifting the probe because this will result in loss of alignment with the tip of the transverse process. Instead, the *needle* should be shifted or repositioned to bring it into alignment with both the ultrasound beam and target. Scouting out the optimal insertion site and trajectory with a local anesthetic infiltration needle is also helpful.
- Correct needle tip placement is indicated by linear spread of injectate in both cranial and caudal directions that lifts erector spinae muscle off the transverse processes.
- Resistance to injection usually signifies that the needle tip is embedded in periosteum. It may be necessary to advance the needle tip slightly deeper off the edge of the transverse process to accurately position it within the fascial plane. A shallow trajectory helps in this regard.

CLINICAL INDICATIONS, CONTRAINDICATIONS, AND CURRENT EVIDENCE

The PECS I and II, SAP, and ESP blocks may be used to provide analgesia of the anterolateral thorax in many different acute and chronic pain scenarios, including postsurgical pain and thoracic trauma. The most common of these are briefly discussed later. There are few absolute contraindications to performing these blocks apart from patient refusal and physical or anatomic barriers to needle insertion. The ESP block may be the most suited to continuous catheter insertion, as the site is distant from the surgical field in most instances. These blocks can be considered in anticoagulated patients if necessary, as the site of needle insertion is relatively shallow and compressible, and hematoma formation is unlikely to have serious consequences. They are most usefully viewed as alternatives to more complex and invasive techniques such as thoracic epidural or paravertebral blocks, especially when these are not feasible or have an unfavorable risk-benefit ratio.

Pectoral I and II blocks

There are limited indications for an isolated PECS I block that only anesthetizes the pectoral muscles; examples include subpectoral implantation of a breast prosthesis or pulse generator. The PECS II block provides additional myocutaneous coverage, particularly into the axilla, and can be used in any surgical procedure on the breast and axillary region. The primary indication for the PECS II block is in breast cancer surgery. It has been shown to provide superior analgesia compared with systemic analgesia alone and seems to be as effective as thoracic paravertebral blocks in this setting [19]. It has also been combined with paravertebral blockade to provide surgical anesthesia for breast surgery [20]. A major advantage over the other regional anesthesia techniques is that the PECS II block can be performed in the supine position. Limitations include surgical concerns regarding needle insertion close to the tumor site (with a possible risk of seeding) and disruption of surgical planes of dissection by the injected fluid. The analgesic benefit may also be marginal for very minor or localized breast surgery.

Other described analgesic indications for PECS I and II blocks include cardiac surgery (both via median sternotomy [21] and minimally invasive approaches [22]), clavicular surgery [23], Port-a-Cath implantation and removal [24], and management of zoster-associated chest wall pain [25].

Serratus anterior plane block

The SAP block has been successfully used to provide analgesia in breast surgery and seems to have similar efficacy compared with PECS II block, despite not targeting the pectoral nerves [26]. The deep variant of the SAP block is preferable if there are surgical concerns regarding disruption of the axillary nodal planes of dissection or if there is postsurgical scarring of the superficial serratus anterior plane [12].

At present most of the randomized controlled trial (RCT) evidence for the SAP block is in thoracic surgery. It provides effective analgesia in video-assisted thoracoscopic surgery (VATS) [27,28] as well as thoracotomy for lung resection [29,30] or minimally invasive cardiac surgery [31]. In one RCT, a single-injection SAP block provided a longer duration of analgesia compared with multilevel intercostal nerve block, although not as long as a single-injection thoracic paravertebral block [31]. This limitation may be overcome by catheter insertion, as indicated by another RCT that found that continuous SAP blockade was as effective as thoracic epidural analgesia following thoracotomy [29].

The SAP block is also a useful option in thoracic trauma, although evidence is limited at present to case reports [32–35]. Advantages over thoracic epidural or paravertebral block include the ability to perform it in the supine position, in the presence of head or spine injuries, multisystem trauma, or coagulopathy. The site of injection does however limit its effectiveness to mainly injuries of the anterolateral chest wall.

Erector spinae plane block

The ESP block has been described in the management of a multitude of painful conditions of the thorax, including breast surgery [36–38], thoracic surgery [39,40], cardiac surgery [41–43], thoracic trauma [44,45], cancer pain [46], and persistent postsurgical pain [47,48]. The chief advantage of the ESP block over the SAP and PECS II block is that the dorsal rami and their branches are blocked, providing coverage of the posterolateral thorax [45,49]. There may also be an additional component of visceral analgesia from blockade of the sympathetic chain, although this has yet to be conclusively demonstrated.

Because the ESP block was only first described in late 2016 [47], RCTs have only recently begun to emerge; the results are highly encouraging. ESP blockade at the T5 level provided superior analgesia compared with systemic analgesia alone in breast surgery [36], although another trial suggested that the PECS II block may be more effective [37]. This may reflect a difference in axillary (T2) coverage and could be addressed by performing the ESP block at a higher vertebral level. Bilateral ESP blocks are highly effective in cardiac surgery, not only providing excellent pain control after median sternotomy but also improving patient-centered outcomes such as time to ambulation and oral intake [41]. Continuous bilateral ESP blockade has shown to be comparable to thoracic epidural analgesia in this setting [42] and may have an important role in enhanced recovery pathways after cardiac surgery [43]. A recent study comparing ESP and SAP blocks in VATS reported that although both were effective, the ESP block provided for lower dynamic pain scores and longer time to first request for analgesia [39]. Finally, as with the SAP block, it is an effective analgesic option in thoracic trauma with few contraindications; in a recently published retrospective cohort study of 79 patients, there was significant improvement in respiratory function following ESP blockade together with hemodynamic stability [44].

CURRENT CONTROVERSIES AND FUTURE CONSIDERATIONS

The mechanism of action of the SAP and ESP block remains controversial, given that some cadaveric studies [18,50] have failed to demonstrate consistent injectate spread to the ventral rami or intercostal nerves that would explain the analgesia observed in clinical practice. This is most likely because of the physical limitations of cadaver models, and additional imaging studies in live subjects [17] may shed light on this area.

It is worth noting that several other ultrasound-guided techniques for thoracic analgesia have been described in recent years, including the retrolaminar block [15,16], the midpoint transverse process to pleura block [51], the rhomboid-intercostal and subserratus plane block [52], and parasternal blocks such as the transversus thoracis plane block [53,54]. Further research is required to determine the place of these techniques in the anesthesiologist's armamentarium of analgesic options. In addition, a transverse (axial) in-plane technique has recently been described for ESP, and further studies are needed to assess its proposed advantages to the initially described parasagittal in-plane technique for ESP [55,56].

The biggest risk associated with these fascial plane blocks at present is that of LAST, with one center reporting a 1.6% incidence [57]. Pharmacokinetic studies will help to further quantify this risk and guide appropriate dosing.

One major limitation of all single-injection techniques is their limited duration of action. It is presently unclear if adjuncts such as dexamethasone or dexmedetomidine will significantly prolong the duration of fascial plane blocks in the same way as other peripheral nerve blocks. Fortunately, the SAP and ESP blocks lend themselves readily to catheter insertion. However, research is needed to determine if programmed intermittent boluses are superior to continuous infusion regimens, as suggested by anecdotal reports [58] and anatomic principles, as well as to define optimal dosing parameters.

SUMMARY

The ultrasound-guided peripheral nerve blocks of the thorax have been enthusiastically embraced principally because they are simple and safe to perform, and thus represent a more accessible alternative to the traditional regional anesthesia options of thoracic epidural and thoracic paravertebral blockade. The preliminary evidence is highly encouraging, and further comparative studies, particularly of the SAP and ESP blocks, are needed to determine if they are equally efficacious. It is possible that they may fall short, given that the very nature of these blocks involves deposition of local anesthetic distant to the desired neural targets. However, even if thoracic epidural and paravertebral blocks prove superior, this will still have to be weighed against the complexity of performance, the demands of postoperative care, secondary failure, and risk of complications and side effects, particularly hypotension.

References

[1] Sakamoto H, Akita K, Sato T. An anatomical analysis of the relationships between the intercostal nerves and the thoracic and abdominal muscles in man. I. Ramification of the intercostal nerves. Acta Anat 1996;156:132–42.

[2] Loukas M, Hullett J, Louis RG, et al. The gross anatomy of the extrathoracic course of the intercostobrachial nerve. Clin Anat 2006;19:106–11.

[3] Woodworth GE, Ivie RMJ, Nelson SM, et al. Perioperative breast analgesia: a qualitative review of anatomy and regional techniques. Reg Anesth Pain Med 2017;42:609–31.

[4] Capek S, Tubbs RS, Spinner RJ. Do cutaneous nerves cross the midline? Clin Anat 2015;28:96–100.

[5] Ford DJ, Raj PP, Singh P, et al. Differential peripheral nerve block by local anesthetics in the cat. Anesthesiology 1984;60:28–33.

[6] Chin KJ, Adhikary SD, Forero M. Understanding ESP and Fascial Plane Blocks: a Challenge to Omniscience. Reg Anesth Pain Med 2018;43:807–8.

[7] Neal JM, Woodward CM, Harrison TK. The American Society of Regional Anesthesia and Pain Medicine Checklist for Managing Local Anesthetic Systemic Toxicity: 2017 Version. Reg Anesth Pain Med 2018;43:150–3.

[8] Rahiri J, Tuhoe J, Svirkis D, et al. Systematic review of the systemic concentrations of local anaesthetic after transversus abdominis plane and rectus sheath block. Br J Anaesth 2017;118:517–26.

[9] Versyck B, Groen G, van Geffen G-J, et al. The pecs anesthetic blockade: a correlation between magnetic resonance imaging, ultrasound imaging, reconstructed cross-sectional anatomy and cross-sectional histology. Clin Anat 2019;32:421–9.

[10] Blanco R, Parras T, McDonnell JG, et al. Serratus plane block: a novel ultrasound-guided thoracic wall nerve block. Anaesthesia 2013;68:1107–13.

[11] Abdallah FW, Cil T, MacLean D, et al. Too Deep or not too deep?: a propensity-matched comparison of the analgesic effects of a superficial versus deep serratus fascial plane block for ambulatory breast cancer surgery. Reg Anesth Pain Med 2018;43:480–7.

[12] Piracha MM, Thorp SL, Puttanniah V, et al. "A tale of two planes": deep versus superficial serratus plane block for postmastectomy pain syndrome. Reg Anesth Pain Med 2017;42:259–62.

[13] Biswas A, Castanov V, Li Z, et al. Serratus plane block: a cadaveric study to evaluate optimal injectate spread. Reg Anesth Pain Med 2018;43:854–8.

[14] Kunigo T, Murouchi T, Yamamoto S, et al. Injection volume and anesthetic effect in serratus plane block. Reg Anesth Pain Med 2017;42:737–40.

[15] Adhikary SD, Bernard S, Lopez H, et al. Erector spinae plane block versus retrolaminar block: a magnetic resonance imaging and anatomical study. Reg Anesth Pain Med 2018;43:756–62.

[16] Yang HM, Choi YJ, Kwon HJ, et al. Comparison of injectate spread and nerve involvement between retrolaminar and erector spinae plane blocks in the thoracic region: a cadaveric study. Anaesthesia 2018;73:1244–50.

[17] Schwartzmann A, Peng P, Maciel MA, et al. Mechanism of the erector spinae plane block: insights from a magnetic resonance imaging study. Can J Anaesth 2018;65:1165–6.
[18] Ivanusic J, Konishi Y, Barrington MJ. A cadaveric study investigating the mechanism of action of erector spinae blockade. Reg Anesth Pain Med 2018;43:567–71.
[19] Versyck B, van Geffen GJ, Chin KJ. Analgesic efficacy of the Pecs II block: a systematic review and meta-analysis. Anaesthesia 2019;74:663–73.
[20] Pawa A, Wight J, Onwochei DN, et al. Combined thoracic paravertebral and pectoral nerve blocks for breast surgery under sedation: a prospective observational case series. Anaesthesia 2018;73:438–43.
[21] Kumar KN, Kalyane RN, Singh NG, et al. Efficacy of bilateral pectoralis nerve block for ultrafast tracking and postoperative pain management in cardiac surgery. Ann Card Anaesth 2018;21:333–8.
[22] Yalamuri S, Klinger RY, Bullock WM, et al. Pectoral fascial (PECS) I and II blocks as rescue analgesia in a patient undergoing minimally invasive cardiac surgery. Reg Anesth Pain Med 2017;42:764–6.
[23] Schuitemaker RJB, Sala-Blanch X, Rodriguez-Pérez CL, et al. The PECS II block as a major analgesic component for clavicle operations: a description of 7 case reports. Rev Esp Anestesiol Reanim 2018;65:53–8.
[24] Munshey F, Ramamurthi RJ, Tsui B. Early experience with PECS 1 block for Port-a-Cath insertion or removal in children at a single institution. J Clin Anesth 2018;49:63–4.
[25] Kim Y-D, Park S-J, Shim J, et al. Clinical usefulness of pectoral nerve block for the management of zoster-associated pain: case reports and technical description. J Anesth 2016;30:1074–7.
[26] Abdallah FW, MacLean D, Madjdpour C, et al. Pectoralis and serratus fascial plane blocks each provide early analgesic benefits following ambulatory breast cancer surgery: a retrospective propensity-matched cohort study. Anesth Analg 2017;125:294–302.
[27] Kim D-H, Oh YJ, Lee JG, et al. Efficacy of ultrasound-guided serratus plane block on postoperative quality of recovery and analgesia after video-assisted thoracic surgery: a randomized, triple-blind, placebo-controlled study. Anesth Analg 2018;126:1353–61.
[28] Park MH, Kim JA, Ahn HJ, et al. A randomised trial of serratus anterior plane block for analgesia after thoracoscopic surgery. Anaesthesia 2018;73:1260–4.
[29] Khalil AE, Abdallah NM, Bashandy GM, et al. Ultrasound-guided serratus anterior plane block versus thoracic epidural analgesia for thoracotomy pain. J Cardiothorac Vasc Anesth 2017;31:152–8.
[30] Saad FS, El Baradie SY, Abdel Aliem MAW, et al. Ultrasound-guided serratus anterior plane block versus thoracic paravertebral block for perioperative analgesia in thoracotomy. Saudi J Anaesth 2018;12:565–70.
[31] Kaushal B, Chauhan S, Saini K, et al. Comparison of the efficacy of ultrasound-guided serratus anterior plane block, pectoral nerves II block, and intercostal nerve block for the management of postoperative thoracotomy pain after pediatric cardiac surgery. J Cardiothorac Vasc Anesth 2019;33:418–25.
[32] Kunhabdulla NP, Agarwal A, Gaur A, et al. Serratus anterior plane block for multiple rib fractures. Pain Physician 2014;17:E651–3.
[33] Fu P, Weyker PD, Webb CAJ. Case report of serratus plane catheter for pain management in a patient with multiple rib fractures and an inferior scapular fracture. A A Case Rep 2017;8:132–5.
[34] Bossolasco M, Bernardi E, Fenoglio LM. Continuous serratus plane block in a patient with multiple rib fractures. J Clin Anesth 2017;38:85–6.
[35] Durant E, Dixon B, Luftig J, et al. Ultrasound-guided serratus plane block for ED rib fracture pain control. Am J Emerg Med 2017;35:197.
[36] Gürkan Y, Aksu C, Kuş A, et al. Ultrasound guided erector spinae plane block reduces postoperative opioid consumption following breast surgery: a randomized controlled study. J Clin Anesth 2018;50:65–8.

[37] Altıparmak B, Korkmaz Toker M, Uysal Aİ, et al. Comparison of the effects of modified pectoral nerve block and erector spinae plane block on postoperative opioid consumption and pain scores of patients after radical mastectomy surgery: a prospective, randomized, controlled trial. J Clin Anesth 2018;54:61–5.
[38] Kimachi PP, Martins EG, Peng P, et al. The erector spinae plane block provides complete surgical anesthesia in breast surgery: a case report. A A Pract 2018;11:186–8.
[39] Gaballah KM, Soltan WA, Bahgat NM. Ultrasound-guided serratus plane block versus erector spinae block for postoperative analgesia after video-assisted thoracoscopy: a pilot randomized controlled trial. J Cardiothorac Vasc Anesth 2019;33(7):1946–53.
[40] Forero M, Rajarathinam M, Adhikary S, et al. Continuous erector spinae plane block for rescue analgesia in thoracotomy after epidural failure: a case report. A A Case Rep 2017;8:254–6.
[41] Krishna SN, Chauhan S, Bhoi D, et al. Bilateral erector spinae plane block for acute post-surgical pain in adult cardiac surgical patients: a randomized controlled trial. J Cardiothorac Vasc Anesth 2019;33:368–75.
[42] Nagaraja PS, Ragavendran S, Singh NG, et al. Comparison of continuous thoracic epidural analgesia with bilateral erector spinae plane block for perioperative pain management in cardiac surgery. Ann Card Anaesth 2018;21:323–7.
[43] Macaire P, Ho N, Nguyen T, et al. Ultrasound-guided continuous thoracic erector spinae plane block within an enhanced recovery program is associated with decreased opioid consumption and improved patient postoperative rehabilitation after open cardiac surgery-a patient-matched, controlled before-and-after study. J Cardiothorac Vasc Anesth 2019;33(6):1659–67.
[44] Adhikary SD, Liu WM, Fuller E, et al. The effect of erector spinae plane (ESP) block on respiratory and analgesic outcomes in multiple rib fractures: a retrospective cohort study. Anaesthesia 2019;74:585–93.
[45] Luftig J, Mantuani D, Herring AA, et al. Successful emergency pain control for posterior rib fractures with ultrasound-guided erector spinae plane block. Am J Emerg Med 2018;36: 1391–6.
[46] Ramos J, Peng P, Forero M. Long-term continuous erector spinae plane block for palliative pain control in a patient with pleural mesothelioma. Can J Anaesth 2018;65:852–3.
[47] Forero M, Adhikary SD, Lopez H, et al. The erector spinae plane block: a novel analgesic technique in thoracic neuropathic pain. Reg Anesth Pain Med 2016;41:621–7.
[48] Forero M, Rajarathinam M, Adhikary S, et al. Erector spinae plane (ESP) block in the management of post thoracotomy pain syndrome: a case series. Scand J Pain 2017;17:325–9.
[49] Muñoz F, Cubillos J, Bonilla AJ, et al. Erector spinae plane block for postoperative analgesia in pediatric oncological thoracic surgery. Can J Anaesth 2017;64:880–2.
[50] Mayes J, Davison E, Panahi P, et al. An anatomical evaluation of the serratus anterior plane block. Anaesthesia 2016;71:1064–9.
[51] Costache I, de Neumann L, Ramnanan CJ, et al. The mid-point transverse process to pleura (MTP) block: a new end-point for thoracic paravertebral block. Anaesthesia 2017;72: 1230–6.
[52] Elsharkawy H, Maniker R, Bolash R, et al. Rhomboid intercostal and subserratus plane block: a cadaveric and clinical evaluation. Reg Anesth Pain Med 2018;43:745–51.
[53] Ueshima H, Otake H. Addition of transversus thoracic muscle plane block to pectoral nerves block provides more effective perioperative pain relief than pectoral nerves block alone for breast cancer surgery. Br J Anaesth 2017;118:439–43.
[54] Fuji S, Roche M, Jones PM, et al. Transversus thoracis muscle plane block in cardiac surgery: a pilot feasibility study. Reg Anesth Pain Med 2019;44:556–60.
[55] Kwon W, Jung K, Bang S. Novel lateral approach for erector spinae plane block: a convenient and safe method. Reg Anesth Pain Med 2019;44:532–4.

[56] Narayanan M, Venkataraju A. Transverse approach to the erector spinae plane block: is there more? Reg Anesth Pain Med 2019;44:529–30.
[57] Tulgar S, Selvi O, Senturk O, et al. Ultrasound-guided erector spinae plane block: indications, complications, and effects on acute and chronic pain based on a single-center experience. Cureus 2019;11:e3815.
[58] de la Cuadra-Fontaine JC, Altermatt FR. Continuous erector spinae plane (ESP) block: optimizing the analgesia technique. J Cardiothorac Vasc Anesth 2018;32:e2–3.

Advances in Anesthesia 37 (2019) 207–228

ADVANCES IN ANESTHESIA

ELSEVIER
MOSBY

Optimal Management of Hypotension During Cesarean Delivery Under Spinal Anesthesia

Jennifer L. Fichter, MD*, Kenneth E. Nelson, MD

Department of Anesthesiology, Wake Forest School of Medicine, 9th Floor Janeway Tower, 1 Medical Center Boulevard, Winston-Salem, NC 27157, USA

Keywords

• Obstetric anesthesia • Cesarean delivery • Spinal hypotension
• Left uterine displacement • Vasopressor choice • Fluid coloading

Key points

- The management of hypotension under spinal anesthesia for cesarean delivery has evolved remarkably, with previous obstetric dogmas being questioned and novel strategies showing success in robust clinical trials.
- Ongoing investigations are showing that aortocaval compression and its clinical ramifications are neither as ubiquitous nor as straightforward as previously thought.
- Phenylephrine administered via infusion is superior to the use of ephedrine in terms of maternal hemodynamic control and neonatal acid-base status.
- Crystalloid coloading, which can be given quickly and facilitates vasopressor administration, is an effective method for the prevention of hypotension under spinal anesthesia.

INTRODUCTION

Spinal anesthesia was first used for cesarean delivery in the United States in 1941 [1]. Since that time, hypotension during neuraxial anesthesia for cesarean delivery has plagued obstetric anesthesia. Without prophylactic treatment, hypotension occurs in up to 80% of patients undergoing spinal anesthesia for cesarean delivery [2]. Spinal hypotension results in decreased uteroplacental blood flow, fetal acidosis, and maternal symptoms such as nausea, vomiting,

Disclosure: The authors have nothing to disclose.

*Corresponding author. *E-mail address:* jfichter@wakehealth.edu

https://doi.org/10.1016/j.aan.2019.08.008

and decreased consciousness [3]. If severe enough, hypotension can lead to complete maternal cardiovascular collapse [4]. As such, finding the solution to spinal anesthesia–induced hypotension has been likened to discovering the Holy Grail of obstetric anesthesia [5,6].

Maternal death from spinal anesthesia is now rare; however, this was a common occurrence just 50 years ago. Holmes [7] titled his 1957 review, "Spinal Analgesia And Caesarean Delivery; Maternal Mortality." Studies around this time focused on the detrimental effects of aortocaval compression from the supine gravid uterus on maternal hemodynamics and fetal status [8,9]. As a result, management strategies largely targeted maternal positioning to relieve vasculature collapse [10]. Early prevention and treatment measures also included increasing maternal blood volume and decreasing venous capacitance, through techniques such as fluid preloading and compression stockings. As the understanding of hypotension during spinal anesthesia has evolved, so has the management, and what were once considered standard management techniques (ie, left uterine tilt, fluid preloading, lower extremity compression) might now be deemed outdated (Table 1).

This review provides an overview of the definition and pathophysiology of spinal anesthesia–induced hypotension, compares strategies for the prevention and treatment of maternal hypotension, and reviews recent literature supporting a conventional approach to management.

HYPOTENSION DURING SPINAL ANESTHESIA

In the absence of a neuraxial-induced sympathectomy, up to 10% of term women experience hypotension in the supine position [11]. This condition results from compression of the inferior vena cava (IVC) by the term gravid uterus when supine [12]. The disorder has been coined supine hypotensive syndrome of pregnancy. Compression of the IVC results in reduced preload and

Table 1
Chronology of selected events in the evolution of the management of spinal-induced hypotension

1935	Angiography first suggests vascular compression in supine parturients
1953	Supine hypotensive syndrome described
1968	Angiography further defines vascular compression in supine parturients
1972	Crawford wedge and concept of 15° lateral tilt developed
1974	Ephedrine shown to be superior to alpha-agonists in pregnant ewes
2002	Systematic review reports ephedrine, compared with phenylephrine, results in decreased fetal pH
2004	Crystalloid coload shown to be superior to crystalloid preload
2010	Phenylephrine preferred vasopressor and studies show benefit of infusion compared with bolus dosing
2015	In first controlled study, norepinephrine is used to adequately maintain maternal CO and SBP
2015	Traditional concept of aortocaval compression challenged by MRI study

Abbreviations: CO, cardiac output; SBP, systolic blood pressure.

increased maternal heart rate via the baroreceptor-mediated reflex. Symptoms commonly include maternal lightheadedness, dizziness, nausea, and general discomfort [13]. At the extreme, maternal and neonatal death have been attributed to supine hypotensive syndrome of pregnancy [14]. Parturients normally have a well-developed collateral venous system, which enables adequate venous return through the azygous, hemiazygos, and ascending lumbar veins in the event of IVC occlusion [15]. However, in patients with supine hypotensive syndrome, venous collateralization and compensatory mechanisms are apparently less effective.

Hypotension during spinal anesthesia may be exaggerated in patients with supine hypotensive syndrome. Such patients experience baseline symptoms from inadequate preload, which can worsen following neuraxial anesthesia. Spinally administered local anesthetics induce a vasomotor sympathectomy, resulting in decreased systemic vascular resistance (SVR) and redistributed blood volume to the splanchnic and lower extremity circulations [16,17]. The degree of hypotension seems proportional to block height and some investigators have used low-dose bupivacaine spinal anesthesia to reduce hemodynamic alterations [18,19]. For cxample, Van de Velde and colleagues [20] showed that the mean lowest systolic blood pressure (SBP) was higher in patients receiving 6.5 mg of hyperbaric intrathecal bupivacaine compared with 9.5 mg (102 $\pm$ 16 mm Hg vs 88 $\pm$ 16 mm Hg; $P < .05$). In addition to causing less vasodilation, a lower block level is less likely to affect cardioaccelerator fibers originating from thoracic spinal levels 1 to 4 [21]. Once cardioaccelerator fibers are blocked, vagal stimulation predominates, potentially resulting in bradycardia. Cardiac output (CO) is directly related to heart rate and so any reduction in heart rate results in a decrease in CO, presuming stroke volume remains constant.

Recent advances in minimally invasive cardiac monitoring have provided additional insight into the hemodynamic effects of spinal anesthesia. Multiple recent trials have made use of continuous CO monitoring and suprasternal ultrasonography to monitor CO under spinal anesthesia. Langesaeter and colleagues [22] were the first to use the LiDCOplus, a minimally invasive hemodynamic monitor, to measure CO, SVR, and SBP in pregnant women undergoing spinal anesthesia for cesarean delivery. The device uses an arterial line to detect arterial waveform changes based on injected lithium concentrations [22,23]. Women were randomized to low-dose or higher-dose (7 mg vs 10 mg, respectively) isobaric bupivacaine (with sufentanil 4 μg) spinal anesthesia and a prophylactic phenylephrine infusion (0.25 μg/kg/min) versus placebo. They showed significantly lower mean differences in SBP and CO changes from baseline after spinal anesthesia within the group receiving low-dose bupivacaine and prophylactic phenylephrine compared with higher-dose bupivacaine and placebo, which is expected given the increased vasodilatory effects from greater amounts of local anesthetic. What was perhaps a more significant finding from this study was the immediate increase in CO and decrease in SVR associated with spinal anesthesia; this effect was present in all patients, regardless of randomization. No significant differences in stroke volume were found between groups, indicating that CO changes were primarily heart rate driven. In patients without minimally invasive monitoring, heart rate is regarded as the best surrogate marker of CO under spinal anesthesia [23]. Because placental circulation and fetal oxygenation depend more on the maintenance of maternal CO than SBP, an anesthetic plan should optimize all hemodynamic variables, not solely SBP [24,25].

Invasive, even minimally invasive, monitoring is rarely required in the obstetric population and is typically reserved for the highest-risk parturients. As a result, most studies on the cardiovascular response to spinal anesthesia focus on the prevention and treatment of hypotension. Hypotension has multiple definitions in the obstetric anesthesia literature. Definitions have included (1) SBP less than 90 mm Hg or less than 100 mm Hg, (2) SBP less than 80% of baseline, and (3) greater than a 25% decrease in SBP from baseline [26–30]. In practice, surveyed anesthesiologists use different SBP thresholds for vasopressor use, with most using a decrease in SBP greater than 20% [31]. This article does not specifically state the definition for hypotension used for each study discussed; however, it is important to note that such heterogeneity can confound study comparisons.

MATERNAL POSITIONING

In the supine position, the gravid uterus completely occludes the IVC. Bieniarz and colleagues [32] used angiography in the 1960s to determine the degree of vasculature collapse and found that both the IVC and the aorta are compressed when a parturient lies supine (see Table 1). Nonanesthetized parturients typically tolerate aortocaval compression well without significant cardiovascular effects as the result of collateral blood flow. However, during neuraxial anesthesia the induced sympathectomy may result in fetal compromise. Crawford and colleagues [33]were among the first anesthesiologists to draw attention to this matter (see Table 1). They examined 150 women undergoing elective cesarean delivery with general anesthesia, tilting 63 of those patients to the right with the use of a 15° rubber wedge. The remaining 87 women were supine. They found a statistically significant difference in mean umbilical artery pH of newborns from the tilted group, 7.31 versus 7.27 in the nontilted group ($P<.001$). Their study conditions are hardly generalizable to contemporary obstetric anesthesia practice. All women had general anesthesia, there was no mention of vasopressor use, and most patients were tilted to the right, per obstetrician preference. However, tilting mothers laterally 15° has essentially remained obstetric anesthesia dogma for decades.

So, should clinicians still be tilting? The 2016 "Practice Guidelines of Obstetric Anesthesia," established by the American Society of Anesthesiologists and the Society for Obstetric Anesthesia and Perinatology, recommends maintaining left lateral tilt until time of delivery [34]. A Cochrane Review performed just 3 years prior showed that, overall, positioning does not affect the incidence of maternal hypotension [35]. Work by Higuchi and colleagues [36] showed the potential reason for this lack of association (see Table 1). They performed abdominal MRI of 10 healthy pregnant and nonpregnant women in 4 different positions: supine and left lateral tilt at 15°, 30°, and 45°. Imaging showed that the IVC was almost completely collapsed by the gravid uterus in supine parturients. Among the parturient group, IVC volume was only significantly different between the supine and 30° and 45° tilt positions, with no difference found between supine and 15° tilt. Imaging also showed no significant difference in aortic volumes in either group, regardless of amount of tilt. This finding suggests that, in nonanesthetized parturients, CO remains stable, whereas cardiac preload may only start to improve when a 30° to 45° angle is assumed.

Thoracic bioimpedance cardiography has been used to continuously monitor CO, stroke volume, and heart rate with position changes in term, nonanesthetized patients with singleton pregnancies [37]. Bamber and colleagues showed that the full left lateral position resulted in the greatest CO. However, the difference compared with other left tilt positions, including 5° and 12.5°, were nonsignificant. Even supine positioning did not result in a significant mean difference in CO [36]. Rees and colleagues [38] similarly studied the effects of extreme positioning on CO, but with patients under spinal anesthesia. However, they did not monitor CO directly but used signs and symptoms suggestive of low CO, such as maternal nausea, vomiting, and bradycardia. Comparing women in complete left lateral position versus 15° of left tilt following spinal anesthesia, they found no significant presumed changes in CO.

Lateral tilt and left uterine displacement are unlikely to independently solve hypotension during spinal anesthesia. Studies show that not only is it ineffective but it is usually applied inaccurately, as shown by Jones and colleagues [39]. They asked anesthetists to estimate the amount of lateral tilt they had applied during elective cesarean deliveries. Estimated tilt ranged from 7° to 35°, whereas measured tilt did not exceed 15°. If the goal is to prevent IVC obstruction and improve cardiac preload, anesthesia providers would have to tilt parturients to at least 30° (Fig. 1). Such a position would be uncomfortable for the patient and inconvenient for the obstetrician (Fig. 2); however, there are case reports of cesarean deliveries performed in the complete lateral position [37,40,41]. For patients with supine hypotensive syndrome of pregnancy, tilt

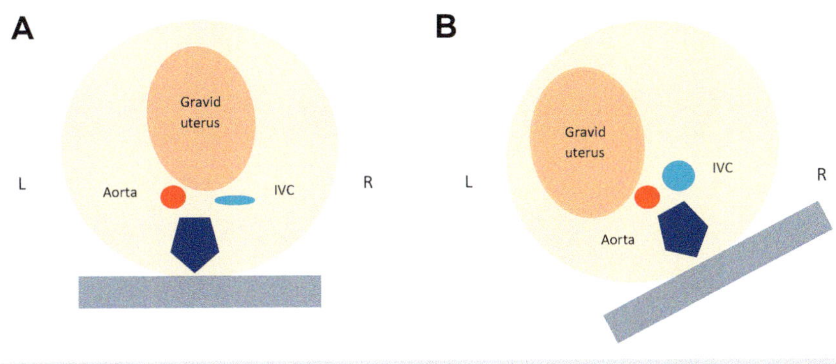

Fig. 1. (*A*) Near-complete IVC occlusion by the gravid uterus in the supine position. (*B*) Relief of IVC occlusion observed at 30° tilt, an angle impractical for cesarean delivery. L, left; R, right.

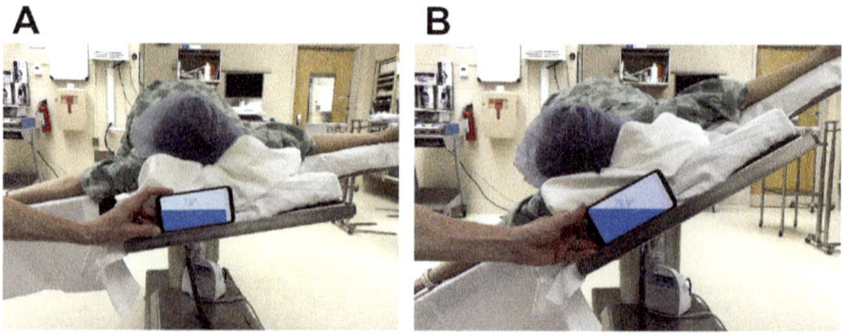

Fig. 2. Maternal positioning during cesarean delivery under spinal anesthesia. (*A*) When positioning the parturient for cesarean delivery following a neuraxial anesthetic, even experienced anesthesia providers typically apply far less than the traditionally recommended 15°. (*B*) The operating room table pictured is maximally tilted with a resulting inclinometer reading of slightly less than 30°. In order to effectively relieve compression of the vena cava, more than 30° of tilt is required, which is poorly tolerated by both patients and surgeons.

should be used. For otherwise asymptomatic parturients, a mild degree of tilt, at the discretion of the anesthesia provider and the obstetrician, may not help but it does not hurt.

EPHEDRINE VERSUS PHENYLEPHRINE

Until a decade or two ago, ephedrine was the preferred vasopressor for the prevention and treatment of spinal-induced hypotension [42]. Early work in pregnant ewes showed improved fetal acidosis when ephedrine was used for hypotension following spinal anesthesia [43]. Compared with pure alpha-agonists, ephedrine caused less vasoconstriction of the uteroplacental circulation, resulting in improved fetal oxygenation [44]. Ephedrine, through indirect beta-agonism, was thought to increase maternal CO and augment uteroplacental blood flow. The use of ephedrine for hypotension was considered gold standard, as shown by surveys of the time. In 1999, 95% of obstetric anesthesiologists in the United Kingdom preferred ephedrine as their sole vasopressor [45]. However, ephedrine's ubiquitous use started to come into question as systematic reviews and later randomized controlled trials unveiled effects on human fetal pH.

In 2002, Lee and colleagues [46] performed a quantitative, systematic review of 7 randomized controlled trials of ephedrine versus phenylephrine given for hypotension for spinal anesthesia during cesarean delivery. When given for the prevention and treatment of hypotension, they found no difference in the incidence of hypotension with the use of ephedrine or phenylephrine (relative risk [RR], 1.0; 95% confidence interval [CI], 0.96–1.06). Limiting analysis to trials specifically of the treatment of hypotension, again, there was no difference between groups. However, they did find statistical significance when comparing umbilical artery pH. Neonates born to mothers receiving phenylephrine had higher umbilical artery pH values (weighted mean difference, 0.03; 95% CI, 0.02–0.04), implying improved uteroplacental perfusion with phenylephrine.

Subsequent prospective studies investigated the effects of phenylephrine, ephedrine, or a combination of the two on maternal cardiovascular and fetal acid-base status. Based on an equipotency ratio of approximately 80:1, phenylephrine 100 μg and ephedrine 5 to 8 mg are typically used for both bolus and infusion dosing [2,47–49]. When administered as a prophylactic bolus dose, ephedrine and phenylephrine show similar efficacy in effectively treating maternal hypotension [47,48]. When used as an infusion, phenylephrine shows superiority over ephedrine. Not only is phenylephrine as an infusion associated with significantly less nausea and vomiting but it more effectively prevents hypotension [49]. More importantly, fewer fetuses are acidotic (pH<7.2) following exposure to phenylephrine versus ephedrine for the management of hypotension following spinal anesthesia.

What this suggests, and what has been supported by additional studies, is that fetal acidosis in the setting of ephedrine use is related to a direct ephedrine effect [50]. Ephedrine stimulates fetal beta-adrenergic receptors, increasing fetal oxygen demand and anaerobic metabolism [51,52]. More often than not, a mixed respiratory and metabolic acidosis results [50]. Although neonatal Apgar scores do not seem to differ between ephedrine and phenylephrine use, studies show increased neonatal complications, such as intraventricular hemorrhage, gastrointestinal dysfunction, and death, in those with metabolic acidosis at birth [53]. As a result, the fetal acidosis observed with ephedrine use has been convincing enough to shift practice to the use of phenylephrine for the prevention and treatment of hypotension following neuraxial anesthesia [47,49–52].

PHENYLEPHRINE INFUSION VERSUS BOLUS

Although phenylephrine is now considered the vasopressor of choice for spinal-induced hypotension during cesarean delivery, the ideal dose and mode of delivery have been debated. Double-blinded studies randomizing patients to either prophylactic phenylephrine infusions or rescue bolus doses have shown conflicting results. In a double-blind, randomized controlled trial of infusion versus the bolus technique, Doherty and colleagues [54] showed improved SBP control in parturients administered phenylephrine boluses. However, this effect was only present within the first 6 minutes after spinal injection and was not deemed clinically significant. The lack of significance may have been the result of the high phenylephrine infusion rate used in the study (120 μg/min). When phenylephrine is delivered at lower infusion rates, this technique may be superior to bolus administration. Siddik-Sayyid and colleagues [55] randomized patients to variable-rate phenylephrine infusions with as-needed boluses versus rescue phenylephrine bolus only. The primary outcome measure was the number of physician interventions to maintain SBP within 20% of baseline. The infusion was initiated at a rate of 0.75 μg/kg/min (equating to 50 μg/min in a 70-kg parturient) immediately after spinal injection and was titrated to maintain goal SBP parameters. The incidence of hypotension was significantly lower in the infusion group, as was the median number of required physician interventions, defined as needing to make any change to the infusion versus giving additional boluses. It must be appreciated that phenylephrine bolus dosing in these studies was performed as treatment of hypotension rather than prophylaxis. In practice, clinicians frequently administer phenylephrine boluses in response to an increase in maternal heart rate, preceding the expected decrease in SBP. Had the infusions been started only after an observed hypotensive episode, the results may have differed significantly.

As a result of ease of delivery and potential hemodynamic benefit, prophylactic phenylephrine infusions have gained favor. The recommended infusion rate ranges from 25 to 50 μg/min, as shown by multiple randomized trials as well as a recently published international consensus statement on the management of hypotension with vasopressors during cesarean section under spinal anesthesia [56]. Compared with higher-dose infusions, with rates reaching 75 to 100 μg/min, low-dose rates equally maintain maternal SBP [57,58]. High-dose infusions may be detrimental to hemodynamic homeostasis. Phenylephrine at fixed rates of 100 μg/min often results in reactive hypertension with additional physician involvement required to reduce blood pressure [58,59]. Such reactive hypertension can precipitate a baroreceptor-mediated bradycardia, which in turn may result in reduced maternal CO.

Investigators have recently used noninvasive monitoring to study specifically the effects of phenylephrine on maternal CO and other hemodynamic parameters. Stewart and colleagues [57] used a handheld suprasternal ultrasonography device to obtain CO measurements in women receiving different rates of phenylephrine (25 μg/min, 50 μg/min, and 100 μg/min) after spinal anesthesia. CO decreased significantly with increasing phenylephrine rate, with a maximum 22% reduction in CO in the group receiving 100 μg/min. Stroke volume remained unchanged in each group. This finding indicates that heart rate changes provide the best indication of CO changes during cesarean delivery under spinal anesthesia [23]. It is important to highlight that most cesarean deliveries during neuraxial anesthesia are performed with the use of noninvasive blood pressure monitoring, and vasopressor choices are based on information obtained from such routine monitors.

SBP is the hemodynamic variable most commonly used as an indicator of adequate hemodynamic control. However, adequate SBP does not necessarily correlate with adequate maternal CO, placental blood flow, and fetal oxygenation. As shown by Stewart and colleagues [57], variable phenylephrine infusion rates provide satisfactory SBP control, but higher rates result in reduced CO. In healthy women with healthy fetuses, a small resultant decrease in CO is unlikely to cause clinically significant effects. However, fetuses with already compromised uteroplacental blood flow may not tolerate additional decreases in perfusion.

It can be concluded that although phenylephrine infusions are effective for maintaining maternal blood pressure and provide an efficient method of vasopressor administration for anesthesia providers, parturient-specific and fetal-specific conditions must be taken into account [60]. In addition, a so-called

Goldilocks approach should be taken when using infusions, using an algorithm as suggested in Fig. 3. A dose high enough to counteract sympathectomy-induced vasodilation, but low enough to avoid excessive vasoconstriction and reduced CO, should be chosen.

OTHER VASOPRESSORS

Ephedrine and phenylephrine are the dominant vasopressors in obstetric anesthesia. At a time when ephedrine was preferred, there was some investigation into infusions of angiotensin II, which seemed promising because it did not result in the tachycardia and fetal acidosis seen with ephedrine use [61]. Although angiotensin II did not gain favor, it showed the benefits of a potential vasopressor that does not affect maternal heart rate and fetal acid-base status. Recently, norepinephrine has shown similar promise [62,63]. Norepinephrine exerts a strong alpha-agonist effect, helping to counteract the decrease in SVR that accompanies spinal anesthesia. Unlike phenylephrine, it has weak beta-adrenergic activity, which promotes positive chronotropy and maintains maternal heart rate and CO. In the treatment of septic shock, norepinephrine is a first-line vasopressor because of evidence showing improved regional and global perfusion, lower lactate concentrations, and improved urine output compared with other vasopressors, including phenylephrine [64]. Although hypotension induced by septic shock and spinal anesthesia differ in pathophysiology, it is worth noting the potential for improved perfusion with norepinephrine use.

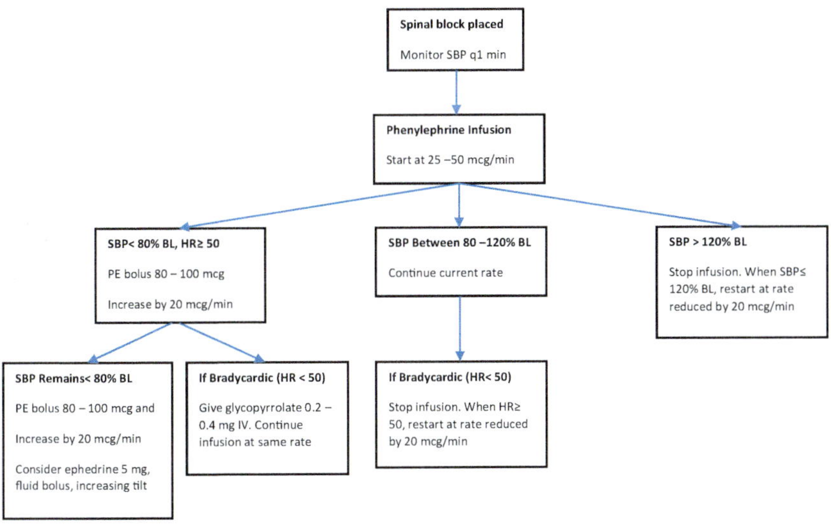

Fig. 3. Phenylephrine infusion titration. Interventions based on changes in SBP every 1 minute. Titration based on work from Refs. [55] and [104]. BL, baseline; HR, heart rate; IV, intravenous; PE, phenylephrine; q, every.

Ngan Kee and colleagues [63] first pioneered work with norepinephrine use in the obstetric population in 2015. Using a norepinephrine to phenylephrine potency ratio of 20:1, they randomized parturients to receive a norepinephrine infusion, rates ranging from 0 to 5 µg/min, or a phenylephrine infusion, rates ranging from 0 to 100 µg/min. At the time of spinal anesthesia for cesarean delivery, patients received a fluid coload and infusion initiation. The infusion was regulated by a computer-controlled, closed-loop feedback system. Although no difference in SBP control was found, patients receiving norepinephrine had significantly greater CO over time (median 102.7% [interquartile ratio (IQR]) 94.3%–116.7%] for norepinephrine vs 93.8% [85.0%–103.1%] for phenylephrine, $P = .004$, median difference 9.8%, 95% CI of difference between medians 2.8%–16.1%). In addition to providing insight into the hemodynamic benefits of norepinephrine, this study suggested that the norepinephrine to phenylephrine potency ratio is lower than 20:1, as previously thought. A potency ratio closer to 13:1 to 16:1 has been suggested by additional work with norepinephrine in the obstetric population [65,66]. In comparison, administering a 100-µg phenylephrine bolus would equate to administering a 6-µg to 8-µg norepinephrine bolus [66].

Subsequent work by Ngan Kee and colleagues [67] showed the efficacy of a manually controlled variable-rate norepinephrine infusion, comparing infusion with bolus norepinephrine use. Parturients receiving norepinephrine via infusion had fewer episodes of hypotension ($P < .001$) compared with those receiving norepinephrine via bolus technique. CO was the same between groups; however, CO values were not available for all study participants. Those receiving norepinephrine as an infusion received an overall higher median rate (dose divided by time to uterine incision) of vasopressor (2.22 µg/min vs 0.28 µg/min) compared with the bolus group. This finding shows that, at low concentrations, at rates much lower than typically used in the intensive care setting, norepinephrine has the potential to effectively decrease the incidence of maternal hypotension during spinal anesthesia.

Obstetric anesthesia providers have expressed some concern regarding norepinephrine use in the obstetric population [62]. This concern arises from systematic reviews and case reports documenting varying degrees of tissue injury following peripheral administration of norepinephrine [68]. However, patients included in these reviews are often septic, have coexisting vascular disease, and require high doses of vasopressor to maintain perfusion. As such, norepinephrine use in healthy parturients is hardly comparable with use in critically ill patients. In addition, norepinephrine used in obstetric studies is formulated in dilute concentrations (5 µg/mL) and is administered at rates much lower than those typically given in the intensive care setting [65,67]. As Carvalho and Dyer [62] suggest, norepinephrine is a promising vasopressor for the management of hypotension during spinal anesthesia. However, before clinicians undergo another paradigm shift in the choice of vasopressor use for cesarean delivery, additional studies will need to confirm norepinephrine's maternal and fetal safety.

FLUID MANAGEMENT

There has been a paradigm shift from ephedrine to phenylephrine use and bolus phenylephrine to infusion phenylephrine use. Fluid type and timing of delivery has also been subject to shifting practice, based on studies of crystalloid versus colloid and fluid preload versus coload. A fluid preload has typically been defined as a bolus of intravenous fluid, ranging from 1 to 2 L, delivered 10 to 20 minutes before spinal anesthesia [69]. A coload is a fluid volume administered immediately after induction of neuraxial anesthesia, and typically completed within 5 minutes [70–72].

PRELOAD VERSUS COLOAD: CRYSTALLOID

Traditional prevention of hypotension during spinal anesthesia supported the use of crystalloid preloading, but studies have failed to show any benefit from this practice [29]. The reason behind this is likely 2-fold. First, crystalloid solutions redistribute from the intravascular to interstitial space within a short period of time. Following a 10-minute infusion of lactated Ringer, less than 50% of the solution is retained with the central compartment at 30 minutes postinfusion [73]. Using indocyanine green concentration to measure blood volume, Ueyama and colleagues [74] showed that only 28% of a lactated Ringer preload infused over 30 minutes remained intravascularly at the end of this half hour. If a preload crystalloid volume is given, by the time a patient experiences sympathectomy-mediated spinal hypotension, most of the crystalloid has already left the intravascular space. Crystalloid preload thus fails to provide additional intravascular volume at the time when it is required to prevent hypotension. Second, any volume load results in atrial stretch, stimulating release of atrial natriuretic peptide (ANP). When a preload is administered, the resulting ANP release induces peripheral vasodilatation and fluid excretion, leading to decreased available intravascular volume coinciding with hypotension from an evolving spinal block [75]. In contrast, coloading provides additional intravascular volume at the time of maximal vasodilatation. When administered concurrently with vasopressors, such as a phenylephrine infusion, a crystalloid coload results in a significantly lower incidence of hypotension (incidence 1.9% [95% CI, 0.3%–9.9%] in phenylephrine/coload group vs 28.3% [95% CI, 18.0%–41.6%] in phenylephrine/minimal fluid maintenance group, $P = .0001$) [59].

PRELOAD VERSUS COLOAD: COLLOID

Colloid coloading has failed to show the benefits found from crystalloid coloading [76]. Colloid preloading has been proposed to increase intravascular volume at a time coinciding with spinal sympathectomy and hypotension better than coloading. Hydroxyethyl starch 6% (HES) has been the most commonly studied colloid in obstetric literature [27,70–72,77–79]. HES and other colloids, such as dextrans, gelatins, and albumin, are large molecules that increase intravascular oncotic pressure and effectively retain plasma volume longer than crystalloid solutions. At 30 minutes after preload with 1.0 L of HES, 100% of colloid has been found to remain within circulation [74]. In a study of 26 parturients undergoing spinal anesthesia for elective cesarean delivery, a 1.0-L HES preload resulted in a significantly lower incidence of hypotension compared with administration of 0.5 L-HES and 1.5-L lactated Ringer preload [74]. When giving HES as a coload, investigators have shown no benefit compared with preloading [70,71]. Other than a significant increase in cardiac output 5 minutes after spinal following an HES preload, Teoh and Sia [70] found no difference in CO at further time points and no difference in SBP at any time. Siddik-Sayyid and colleagues [71] confirmed these results, finding no difference in the incidence of hypotension, severe hypotension (defined as SBP<80 mm Hg), or total amount of vasopressor required following spinal anesthesia. The lack of observed hemodynamic benefit from preloaded HES may be explained again by the release of ANP. Any potential increase in plasma volume from colloid administration may be offset by resultant vasodilation and natriuresis.

VARIED FLUID PRELOADING VERSUS COLOADING COMBINATIONS

Additional studies have investigated the effects of various combinations of fluid type and timing. Tamilselvan and colleagues [78] conducted a double-blind, randomized controlled study of the hemodynamic impact of fluid type given before spinal anesthesia for elective cesarean delivery. A crystalloid solution (Hartmann solution) 1.5 L or 6% HES 0.5 or 1.0 L were delivered 30 minutes before combined spinal-epidural anesthesia. Cardiac parameters were measured with the use of suprasternal ultrasonography throughout this period. Although there was no significant difference in the incidence of hypotension between fluid groups, the study was underpowered for this specific outcome. However, CO remained significantly higher than baseline in the 20 minutes postspinal only in the group receiving HES 1.0 L [78]. For elective cesarean deliveries, clinicians potentially have time to preload patients a half hour before anesthesia. However, this approach is impractical for the large percentage of cesarean deliveries that are unplanned. Coloading can be given quickly and can help deliver concurrently administered vasopressors. McDonald and colleagues [72] randomized patients to a coload of HES 1.0 L or Hartmann solution in addition to a phenylephrine infusion set at 100 μg/min, initiated at the time of spinal injection. Postspinal, the incidence of hypotension was the same between groups and there were no between-group differences in CO. When given as a coload, colloid likely has no advantage over crystalloid.

When given as a preload, colloids may confer some benefit over crystalloid. However, HES 6% (hetastarch), the colloid most researched in the obstetric literature, is no longer routinely available and so future research endeavors will need to study the potential benefits of colloid alternatives. For example, human albumin has not been extensively studied in the obstetric population but may be a viable colloid option for hypotension management and an area for future research. In the interim, hypotension during spinal anesthesia can be efficiently and effectively managed with a 1-L to 2-L crystalloid coload, initiated at the time of spinal block placement and administered over approximately 5 minutes. Not only does this increase intravascular volume at the time of maximal sympathectomy but it facilitates the delivery of concurrently given vasopressors.

SEROTONIN ANTAGONISTS

Although the major cause of hypotension following spinal anesthesia is secondary to sympathetic blockade, the Bezold-Jarisch reflex (BJR) may also contribute to cardiovascular instability. This reflex causes a triad of vasodilation, bradycardia, and hypotension [79]. Stimulation of receptors in the ventricular walls (mechanoreceptors and chemoreceptors) has been implicated in the BJR. In response to decreased venous return, intracardiac mechanoreceptors are stimulated, resulting in cardiac afferent fiber activation and bradycardia. Such bradycardia may be protective, enabling increased diastolic filling time during a period of reduced preload [80]. Chemoreceptors responding to 5-hydroxytryptamine3 (5-HT3 [serotonin]) also contribute to the BJR, as shown by inhibition of the reflex with the use of 5-HT3 antagonists in animal models [81,82]. Animal model results have subsequently been replicated in humans. Results from 2 recent meta-analyses suggest that the use of prophylactic 5-HT3 receptor antagonists reduces the incidence of hypotension during spinal anesthesia [83,84]. Both meta-analyses included randomized controlled trials from the obstetric and nonobstetric populations. Subgroup analyses on the obstetric populations showed significantly lower incidences of hypotension, bradycardia, and nausea/vomiting. For the prevention of hypotension and bradycardia, the number needed to treat was 5.3 and 7.6, respectively [83]. Ondansetron was the most frequently used 5-HT3 antagonist; however, granisetron was given in one obstetric randomized controlled trial.

Although it seems that 5-HT3 antagonists play a role in the prevention of spinal-induced hypotension, there is a large amount of heterogeneity and some degree of publication bias within these analyses [84]. The high heterogeneity was related to the differences in spinal medication, vasopressor use, and fluid management. Half of the obstetric trials included in the Heesen and colleagues[83] analysis used ephedrine as the pressor of choice, making such results less applicable to recommended practice with phenylephrine use. A recent study by Karacaer and colleagues [85] investigated the effect of ondansetron as part of an anesthetic that more fully embraces current accepted practice. Patients scheduled for elective cesarean delivery received a crystalloid coload and norepinephrine 5-μg boluses for refractory hypotension. A prophylactic 8-mg dose of ondansetron compared with saline placebo did not reduce the incidence of hypotension. However, it did result in a significantly lower requirement for norepinephrine ($P = .009$).

Should all parturients undergoing spinal anesthesia for cesarean delivery receive 5-HT3 antagonists? There are not enough prospective data to conclude that higher doses (eg, 8 mg of ondansetron) of 5-HT3 antagonists prevent hypotension during spinal anesthesia for cesarean delivery. With regard to administering 4 mg of ondansetron, providing such low doses is unlikely to cause harm and may help prevent maternal nausea and vomiting during spinal anesthesia for cesarean delivery [83,84].

LOWER EXTREMITY MANIPULATION

The goal of lower extremity manipulation, via leg compression or elevation, is to increase venous return to the central circulation following spinal-induced sympathectomy [86]. Studies have investigated lower extremity elevation and various methods of mechanical compression, including elastic bandages, sequential compression devices, and thromboembolic deterrent stockings, to prevent hypotension following spinal anesthesia [87–91]. Of these studies, Rout and colleagues [91] enrolled one of the largest groups of parturients. They randomized 97 parturients undergoing elective cesarean delivery with spinal anesthesia to 1 of 3 interventions: leg elevation to 30°, leg elevation plus wrapping with elastic bandages, or no elevation with sham bandages (control). Compared with the control group, the leg-wrapped group showed a 5-fold decrease in the incidence of hypotension (odds ratio [OR], 5.3; 95% CI, 1.7–16.3). Leg elevation seemed to have no influence on hypotension.

Although other investigators have shown similar moderate success with lower extremity manipulation, the benefit remains controversial. A recent Cochrane Review analyzed 11 studies with a total of 705 women, comparing lower limb compression with control. Compression prevented hypotension after spinal anesthesia with an average RR of 0.61 (95% CI, 0.47–0.78; $I2 = 65\%$); however, the review deemed the evidence as overall very low quality [92]. In addition, many of the included studies used fluid preloading and ephedrine as the primary vasopressor, making them less comparable with recommended practice. Kuhn and colleagues [93] addressed this issue by performing a randomized, double-blinded, placebo-controlled study in which women undergoing elective cesarean delivery received phenylephrine, leg wrapping, or no treatment under spinal anesthesia. Every patient received a 1-L coload and those randomized to phenylephrine received a 0.25-μg/kg bolus followed by 0.25-μg/kg/min infusion at the time of spinal block. Study design included the LiDCOplus monitor, enabling continuous hemodynamic monitoring of CO and SVR. The phenylephrine group experienced significantly less hypotension compared with the leg-wrapping and control groups. Although continuous CO was reduced in those receiving phenylephrine, SVR was significantly higher in this group. In addition, a rapid and profound reduction in SVR preceded a decrease in blood pressure in all 3 groups, confirming that a sudden and marked arterial vasodilatation is the main hemodynamic effect of spinal anesthesia. The decrease in SVR was only attenuated by phenylephrine, which highlights that leg wrapping does not counteract arterial dilatation. Thus, the prophylactic alpha-1 agonist action of phenylephrine is the more physiologic approach to prevention of spinal-induced hypotension.

For elective, low-risk cesarean deliveries in which this is no time constraint, lower extremity compression devices can be considered. Although they are unlikely to significantly prevent hypotension during spinal anesthesia, leg wrapping may provide some additional preload. For urgent or emergent deliveries, leg compression is an unnecessary component of hypotension management, given the availability of vasopressors and fluid coloading, which are more likely to effectively and efficiently prevent and treat hemodynamic instability.

HYPOTENSION MANAGEMENT IN NONELECTIVE, HIGH-RISK PREGNANCIES

Most studies investigating hypotension following spinal anesthesia have been performed in low-risk parturients undergoing elective, primary cesarean deliveries. As such, obstetric anesthesia has developed gold standards of hypotension management based on healthy mothers and fetuses. It is important to question whether such standards of care are appropriate, for example, for parturients with cardiac disease or with growth-restricted fetuses. In a retrospective observational study of 385 parturients having spinal anesthesia for high-risk cesarean deliveries, there was no statistical difference in fetal pH between patients receiving ephedrine, phenylephrine, or no vasopressor for prophylaxis and treatment of hypotension [51]. High-risk deliveries were defined as cesarean deliveries for pregnancy-induced hypertension, prolonged rupture of membranes, cord prolapse, dystocia, and nonreassuring fetal heart tracings. This lack of difference in fetal pH may be caused by the lower median dose of ephedrine administered, 12 mg (IQR, 6–18 mg) before delivery, compared with doses given in studies of low-risk, elective cesarean deliveries [49,51,94]. Prospective, randomized controlled trials have shown similar findings. In a study of emergency cesarean deliveries under spinal anesthesia performed for acute fetal compromise, Jain and colleagues [95] showed no difference in fetal acidosis between women receiving ephedrine or phenylephrine (umbilical artery pH <7.2, 31.1% in ephedrine group and 20% in phenylephrine group; $P = .22$).

The lack of difference in fetal acidosis between parturients receiving ephedrine and phenylephrine may also be explained by the fact that many women undergoing nonelective cesarean deliveries are laboring. The earliest study describing this effect was performed by Clark and colleagues [96]. They found that healthy women in early labor undergoing cesarean delivery with spinal anesthesia had a significantly lower rate of hypotension compared with nonlaboring women ($P<.05$). It was proposed that uterine contractions delivering additional blood volume to the central compartment contributed to this effect.

Patients with hypertensive disorders of pregnancy have also been shown to require less vasopressor for the treatment of hypotension from spinal anesthesia [97]. Studies within this patient population are limited, but evidence from prospective trials shows this association. Aya and colleagues [98] performed the first study of the incidence of spinal-induced hypotension in preeclamptic compared with healthy parturients. They showed a significantly lower risk of hypotension in patients with preeclampsia with severe features undergoing spinal anesthesia for scheduled cesarean delivery compared with normotensive parturients (OR, 0.17; 95% CI, 0.05–0.58; $P = .006$) and proposed that this is caused by the underlying pathophysiology of the disease. Preeclampsia results in altered vascular endothelium, decreased vascular tone regulation, and increased sympathetic activity [99,100]. As a result, preeclamptic patients may be less susceptible to the sudden decrease in sympathetic tone related to spinal anesthesia.

For preeclamptic patients, clinicians can expect to see less hypotension during spinal anesthesia and potentially a greater effect from vasopressor use. As Sharwood and colleagues[101] also proposed, preeclamptic patients are less dependent on sympathetic output and are potentially more sensitive to sympathomimetic medications. Should preeclamptic patients require vasopressor support, either phenylephrine or ephedrine can be considered, with care taken to carefully titrate so as not to cause iatrogenic hypertension. Fluid delivery in this patient population should also be conservative. Preeclamptic patients are less likely to require a 1-L to 2-L crystalloid coload and delivery of such fluid may potentially lead to volume overload.

SUMMARY AND FUTURE DIRECTIONS

Over the past several decades, the subspecialty of obstetric anesthesia has witnessed a progressive evolution in the management of hypotension with spinal anesthesia during cesarean delivery. The work of dedicated researchers has provided insight into the pathophysiology, the consequences, and the optimal prevention and treatment of maternal hypotension. Current recommended practices for the prevention of hypotension during spinal anesthesia are outlined in Fig. 4. Such practices include administration of 1 to 2 L of crystalloid

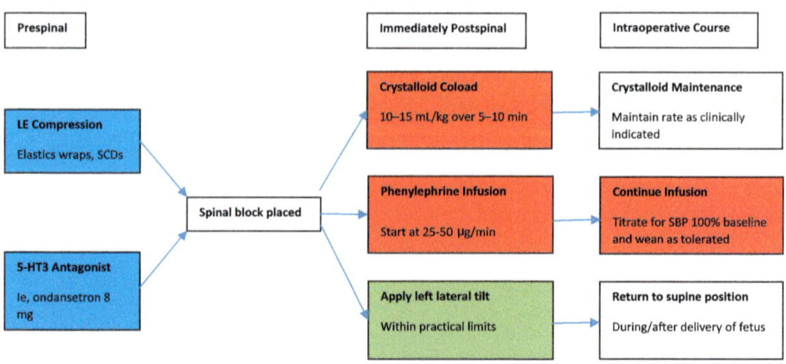

Fig. 4. Management techniques for prevention of hypotension under spinal anesthesia. Code color represents level of recommended implementation: red, high; green, moderate; blue, low. LE, lower extremity; SCD, sequential compression device.

as a coload (or 500 mL of 0.5-L to 1.0-L colloid preload, time permitting) and initiation of a phenylephrine infusion of 25 to 50 μg/min at the time of spinal block placement. Lateral tilt may or may not be used, depending on the presence of preexisting supine hypotension of pregnancy and the response to the measures discussed earlier, keeping in mind that there are few disadvantages to continuing the practice of routinely tilting parturients [102–104]. The treatment of hypotension should include vasopressor infusion titration to maintain SBP near baseline, while ensuring that reactive hypertension does not occur.

Although conventional management prevents and treats hypotension in most patients, clinicians should continue to strive for successful management in every patient. Future work will help to fine tune the current standard practice. Such fine-tuning is likely to include methods to maintain maternal CO rather than SBP, given evidence that placental blood flow depends more on CO than systolic pressure [23]. The advent of minimally invasive and noninvasive cardiac monitoring, such as LiDCOplus, thoracic bioimpedance, and suprasternal cardiac ultrasonography, and their validation in the obstetric population, have provided the opportunity to continuously monitor maternal CO. The growth of point-of-care ultrasonography will also make it possible to titrate fluids and vasopressors based on cardiac filling and function. Perhaps 5-HT3 antagonists will be shown to provide consistent additional benefit, particularly in patients who may be susceptible to the BJR following spinal anesthesia. Norepinephrine infusions might become routinely adopted as concerns regarding the safety of peripheral intravenous administration are fully addressed. Obstetric anesthesia is entering an era in which delivery of care will not only be further optimized but individualized for each mother and her baby.

References

[1] DeCarle DW. Spinal anesthesia in cesarean section. JAMA 1954;154(7):545–9.
[2] Saravanan S, Kocarev M, Wilson RC, et al. Equivalent dose of ephedrine and phenylephrine in the prevention of post-spinal hypotension in caesarean section. Br J Anaesth 2006;96:95–9.
[3] Marx GF, Cosmi EV, Wollman SB. Biochemical status and clinical condition of mother and infant at cesarean section. Anesth Analg 1969;48:986–93.
[4] Comito C, Bechi L, Serena C, et al. Cardiac arrest in the delivery room after spinal anesthesia for cesarean section: a case report and review of literature. J Matern Fetal Neonatal Med 2018;1–3; https://doi.org/10.1080/14767058.2018.1517321.
[5] Macarthur A. Solving the problem of spinal-induced hypotension in obstetric anesthesia. Can J Anaesth 2002;49:536–9.
[6] Campbell JP, Stocks GM. Management of hypotension with vasopressors at cesarean section under spinal anesthesia-have we found the holy grail of obstetric anesthesia? Anaesthesia 2018;73:3–6.
[7] Holmes F. Spinal analgesia and caesarean section; maternal mortality. J Obstet Gynaecol Br Emp 1957;64:229–32.
[8] Ang CK, Tan TH, Walters WA, et al. Postural influence on maternal capillary oxygen and carbon dioxide tension. BMJ 1969;3:201.
[9] Goodlin RC. Aortocaval compression during cesarean section. Obstet Gynecol 1971;37:702.

[10] Colon-Morales MA. A self-supporting device for continuous left uterine displacement during cesarean section. Anesth Analg 1970;49:223.
[11] Howard BK, Goodson JH, Mengert WE. Supine hypotensive syndrome in late pregnancy. Obstet Gynecol 1953;1:371–7.
[12] Humphries A, Ali Mirjalili SA, Tarr GP, et al. The effect of supine positioning on maternal hemodynamics during late pregnancy. J Matern Fetal Neonatal Med 2018;1–8; https://doi.org/10.1080/14767058.2018.1478958.
[13] Lanni SM, Tillinghast J, Silver HM. Hemodynamic changes and baroreflex gain in the supine hypotensive syndrome. Am J Obstet Gynecol 2002;187:1636–41.
[14] De-Giorgio F, Grassi VM, Vetrugno G, et al. Supine hypotensive syndrome as the probable cause of both maternal and fetal death. J Forensic Sci 2012;57:1646–9.
[15] Golub RM, Parsons RE, Sigel B, et al. A review of venous collaterals in inferior vena cava obstruction. Clin Anat 1992;5:441–51.
[16] Mueller RP, Lynn RB, Sancetta SM, et al. Studies of hemodynamic changes in humans following induction of low and high spinal anesthesia. II. The changes in splanchnic blood flow, oxygen extraction and consumption, and splanchnic vascular resistance in humans not undergoing surgery. Circulation 1952;6:894–901.
[17] Tihtonen K, Koobi T, Yli-Hankala A, et al. Maternal hemodynamics during cesarean delivery assessed by whole-body impedance cardiography. Acta Obstet Gynecol Scand 2005;84:355–61.
[18] Leo S, Sng BL, Lim Y, et al. A randomized comparison of low doses of hyperbaric bupivacaine in combined spinal-epidural anesthesia for cesarean delivery. Anesth Analg 2009;109:1600–5.
[19] Teoh WH, Thomas E, Tan HM. Ultra-low dose combined spinal-epidural anesthesia with intrathecal bupivacaine 3.75mg for cesarean delivery: a randomized controlled trial. Int J Obstet Anesth 2006;15:273–8.
[20] Van de Velde M, Van Schoutbroeck D, Jani J, et al. Combined spinal epidural anesthesia for cesarean section: dose dependent effects of hyperbaric bupivacaine on maternal hemodynamics. Anesth Analg 2006;103:187–90.
[21] Miller RD. Miller's anesthesia. 8th edition. Philadelphia: Churchill Livingstone/Elsevier; 2015.
[22] Langesaeter E, Rosseland LA, Stubhaug A. Continuous invasive blood pressure and cardiac output monitoring during cesarean delivery. Anesthesiology 2008;109:856–63.
[23] Dyer RA, Reed AR, van Dyk D, et al. Hemodynamic effects of ephedrine, phenylephrine, and the coadministration of phenylephrine with oxytocin during spinal anesthesia for elective cesarean delivery. Anesthesiology 2009;111:753–65.
[24] Skjoldebrand A, Eklund J, Johansson H, et al. Uteroplacental blood flow measured by placental scintigraphy during epidural anaesthesia for caesarean section. Acta Anaesthesiol Scand 1990;34:79–84.
[25] Sharkey AM, Siddigui N, Downey K, et al. Comparison of intermittent intravenous boluses of phenylephrine and norepinephrine to prevent and treat spinal-induced hypotension in cesarean deliveries: randomized controlled trial. Anesth Analg 2018. [Epub ahead of print].
[26] Calvache JA, Munoz MF, Baron FJ. Hemodynamic effects of a right lumbar-pelvic wedge during spinal anesthesia for cesarean section. Int J Obstet Anesth 2011;20:307–11.
[27] Tawfik MM, Hayes SM, Jacoub FY, et al. Comparison between colloid preload and crystalloid co-load in cesarean section under spinal anesthesia: a randomized controlled trial. Int J Obstet Anesth 2014;23:317–23.
[28] Kaufner L, Karekla A, Henkelmann A, et al. Crystalloid coloading vs. colloid coloading in elective Caesarean section: postspinal hypotension and vasopressor consumption, a prospective, observational clinical trial. J Anesth 2019;33:40–9.

[29] Dyer RA, Farina Z, Joubert IA, et al. Crystalloid preload versus rapid crystalloid administration after induction of spinal anaesthesia (coload) for elective caesarean section. Anaesth Intensive Care 2004;32:351–7.
[30] Ngan Kee WD. Prevention of maternal hypotension after regional anaesthesia for caesarean section. Curr Opin Anaesthesiol 2010;23:304–9.
[31] Allen TK, Muir HA, George RB, et al. A survey of the management of spinal-induced hypotension for scheduled cesarean delivery. Int J Obstet Anesth 2009;18:356–61.
[32] Bieniarz J, Crottogini JJ, Curuchet E, et al. Aortocaval compression by the uterus in late pregnancy: II. An arteriographic study. Am J Obstet Gynecol 1968;100:203–17.
[33] Crawford JS, Burton M, Davies P. Time and lateral tilt at Caesarean section. Br J Anaesth 1972;44:477–84.
[34] Practice guidelines for obstetric anesthesia: An updated report by the American Society of Anesthesiologists Task Force on Obstetric Anesthesia and the Society for Obstetric Anesthesia and Perinatology. Anesthesiology 2016;124:270–300.
[35] Cluver C, Novikova N, Hofmeyr GJ, et al. Maternal position during caesarean section for preventing maternal and neonatal complications. Cochrane Database Syst Rev 2013;28: 1–44.
[36] Higuchi H, Takagi S, Zhang K, et al. Effect of lateral tilt angle on the volume of the abdominal aorta and inferior vena cava in pregnant and nonpregnant women determined by magnetic resonance imaging. Anesthesiology 2015;122:286–93.
[37] Bamber JH, Dresner M. Aortocaval compression in pregnancy: The effect of changing the degree and direction of lateral tilt on maternal cardiac output. Anesth Analg 2003;97: 256–8.
[38] Rees SG, Thurlow JA, Gardner IC, et al. Maternal cardiovascular consequences of positioning after spinal anaesthesia for Caesarean section: Left 15-degree table tilt vs. left lateral. Anaesthesia 2002;57:15–20.
[39] Jones SJ, Kinsella SM, Donald FA. Comparison of measured and estimated angles of table tilt at Caesarean section. Br J Anaesth 2003;90:86–7.
[40] Waldron KW, Wood C. Cesarean section in the lateral position. Obstet Gynecol 1971;37:706–10.
[41] Coffman JC, Legg RL, Coffman CF, et al. Lateral position for cesarean delivery because of severe aortocaval compression in a patient with Marfan Syndrome: a case report. A A Case Rep 2017;8:93–5.
[42] Morgan P. The role of vasopressors in the management of hypotension induced by spinal and epidural anaesthesia. Can J Anaesth 1994;41:404–13.
[43] Shnider S, DeLorimier AA, Holl JW, et al. Vasopressors in obstetrics: I. Correction of fetal acidosis with ephedrine during spinal hypotension. Am J Obstet Gynecol 1968;102: 911–9.
[44] Ralston DH, Shnider SM, DeLorimier AA. Effects of equipotent ephedrine, metaraminol, mephentermine, and methoxamine on uterine blood flow in the pregnant ewe. Anesthesiology 1974;40:354–70.
[45] Burns SM, Cowan CM, Wilkes RG. Prevention and management of hypotension during spinal anaesthesia for elective Caesarean section: a survey of practice. Anaesthesia 2001;56:794–8.
[46] Lee A, Ngan Kee WD, Gin T. A quantitative, systemic review of randomized controlled trials of ephedrine versus phenylephrine for the management of hypotension during spinal anesthesia for cesarean delivery. Anesth Analg 2002;94:920–6.
[47] Prakash S, Pramanik V, Chellani H, et al. Maternal and neonatal effects of bolus administration of ephedrine and phenylephrine during spinal anaesthesia for caesarean delivery: a randomized study. Int J Obstet Anesth 2010;19:24–30.
[48] Thomas DG, Robson SC, Redfern H, et al. Randomized trial of bolus phenylephrine or ephedrine for maintenance of arterial pressure during spinal anaesthesia for Caesarean section. Br J Anaesth 1996;76:61–5.

[49] Ngan Kee WD, Lee A, Khaw KS, et al. A randomized double-blinded comparison of phenylephrine and ephedrine infusion combinations to maintain blood pressure during spinal anesthesia for cesarean delivery: the effects on fetal acid-base status and hemodynamic control. Anesth Analg 2008;107:1295–302.
[50] Cooper DW, Carpenter M, Mowbray P, et al. Fetal and maternal effects of phenylephrine and ephedrine during spinal anesthesia for cesarean delivery. Anesthesiology 2002;97:1582–90.
[51] Cooper DW, Sharma S, Orakkan P, et al. Retrospective study of association between choice of vasopressor given during spinal anaesthesia for high-risk caesarean delivery and fetal pH. Int J Obstet Anesth 2010;19:44–9.
[52] Ngan Kee WD, Khaw KS, Tan PE, et al. Placental transfer and fetal metabolic effects of phenylephrine and ephedrine during spinal anesthesia for cesarean delivery. Anesthesiology 2009;111:506–12.
[53] Low JA, Panagiotopoulos C, Derrick EJ. Newborn complications after intrapartum asphyxia with metabolic acidosis in the term fetus. Am J Obstet Gynecol 1994;170:1081–7.
[54] Doherty A, Ohashi Y, Downey K, et al. Phenylephrine infusion versus bolus regimens during cesarean delivery under spinal anesthesia: a double-blind randomized clinical trial to assess hemodynamic changes. Anesth Analg 2012;115:1343–50.
[55] Siddik-Sayyid SM, Taha SK, Kanazi GE, et al. A randomized controlled trial of variable rate phenylephrine infusion with rescue phenylephrine boluses versus rescue boluses alone on physician interventions during spinal anesthesia for elective cesarean delivery. Anesth Analg 2014;118:611–8.
[56] Kinsella SM, Carvalho B, Dyer RA, et al. International consensus statement on the management of hypotension with vasopressors during cesarean section under spinal anesthesia. Anaesthesia 2018;73:71–92.
[57] Stewart A, Fernando R, McDonald S, et al. The dose-dependent effects of phenylephrine for elective cesarean delivery under spinal anesthesia. Anesth Analg 2010;111:1230–7.
[58] Allen TK, George RB, White WD, et al. A double-blind, placebo-controlled trial of four fixed rate infusion regimens of phenylephrine for hemodynamic support during spinal anesthesia for cesarean delivery. Anesth Analg 2010;111:1221–9.
[59] Ngan Kee WD, Khaw KS, Ng FF. Prevention of hypotension during spinal anesthesia for cesarean delivery: an effective technique using combination phenylephrine infusion and crystalloid cohydration. Anesthesiology 2005;103:744–50.
[60] Ngan Kee WD. Phenylephrine infusions for maintaining blood pressure during spinal anesthesia for cesarean delivery: finding the shoe that fits. Anesth Analg 2014;118:496–8.
[61] Vincent RD, Werhan CF, Norman PF, et al. Prophylactic angiotensin II infusion during spinal anesthesia for elective cesarean delivery. Anesthesiology 1998;88:1475–9.
[62] Carvalho B, Dyer RA. Norepinephrine for spinal hypotension during cesarean delivery: another paradigm shift? Anesthesiology 2015;122:728–30.
[63] Ngan Kee WD, Lee SW, NG FF, et al. Randomized double-blinded comparison of norepinephrine and phenylephrine for maintenance of blood pressure during spinal anesthesia for cesarean delivery. Anesthesiology 2015;122:736–45.
[64] Avni T, Lador A, Lev S, et al. Vasopressors for the treatment of septic shock: systematic review and meta-analysis. PLoS One 2015;10:e0129305.
[65] Ngan Kee WD. A random-allocation graded dose-response study of norepinephrine and phenylephrine for treating hypotension during spinal anesthesia for cesarean delivery. Anesthesiology 2017;127:934–41.
[66] Onwochei DN, Ngan Kee WD, Fung L, et al. Norepinephrine intermittent intravenous boluses to prevent hypotension during spinal anesthesia for cesarean delivery: a sequential allocation dose-finding study. Anesth Analg 2017;125:212–8.

[67] Ngan Kee WD, Lee SWY, Ng FF, et al. Prophylactic norepinephrine infusion for preventing hypotension during spinal anesthesia for cesarean delivery. Anesth Analg 2018;126: 1989–94.
[68] Loubani OM, Green RS. A systematic review of extravasation and local tissue injury from administration of vasopressors through peripheral intravenous catheters and central venous catheters. J Crit Care 2015;30:653.e9-17.
[69] Jackson R, Reid JA, Thorburn J. Volume preloading is not essential to prevent spinal-induced hypotension at Caesarean section. Br J Anaesth 1995;75:262–5.
[70] Teoh WH, Sia AT. Colloid preload versus coload for spinal anesthesia for cesarean delivery: the effects on maternal cardiac output. Anesth Analg 2009;108:1592–8.
[71] Siddik-Sayyid SM, Nasr VG, Taha SK, et al. A randomized trial comparing colloid preload to coload during spinal anesthesia for elective cesarean delivery. Anesth Analg 2009;109:1219–24.
[72] McDonald S, Fernando R, Ashpole K, et al. Maternal cardiac output changes after crystalloid or colloid coload following spinal anesthesia for elective cesarean delivery: a randomized controlled trial. Anesth Analg 2011;113:803–10.
[73] Svensen C, Rodhe PM, Olsson J, et al. Arteriovenous differences in plasma dilution and the distribution kinetics of lactated Ringer's solution. Anesth Analg 2009;108:128–33.
[74] Ueyama H, He YL, Tanigami H, et al. Effects of crystalloid and colloid preload on blood volume in the parturient undergoing spinal anesthesia for elective cesarean section. Anesthesiology 1999;91:1571–6.
[75] Pouta AM, Karinen J, Vuolteenaho OJ, et al. Effect of intravenous fluid preload on vasoactive peptide secretion during caesarean section under spinal anaesthesia. Anaesthesia 1996;51:128–32.
[76] Carvalho B, Mercier FJ, Riley ET, et al. Hetastarch co-loading is as effective as preloading for the prevention of hypotension following spinal anaesthesia for caesarean delivery. Int J Obstet Anesth 2009;18:150–5.
[77] Arora P, Singh RM, Kundra S, et al. Fluid administration before caesarean delivery: does type and timing matter? J Clin Diagn Res 2015;9:UC01–4.
[78] Tamilselvan P, Fernando R, Bray J, et al. The effects of crystalloid and colloid preload on cardiac output in the parturient undergoing planned cesarean delivery under spinal anesthesia: a randomized trial. Anesth Analg 2009;109:1916–21.
[79] Campagna JA, Carter C. Clinical relevance of the Bezold-Jarisch reflex. Anesthesiology 2003;98:48–58.
[80] Sander-Jensen K, Marving J, Secher NH, et al. Does the decrease in heart rate prevent a detrimental decrease of the end-systolic volume during central hypovolemia in man? Angiology 1990;41:687–95.
[81] Yamano M, Ito H, Kamato T, et al. Characteristics of inhibitory effects of serotonin (5-HT)3-receptor antagonists, YM060 and YM114 (KAE-393), on the von Bezold-Jarisch reflex induced by 2-Methyl-5HT, veratridine and electrical stimulation of vagus nerves in anesthetized rats. Jpn J Pharmacol 1995;69:351–6.
[82] Yamano M, Kamato T, Nishida A, et al. Serotonin (5-HT)3-receptor antagonism of 4,5,6,7-tetrahydrobenzimidazole derivatives against 5-HT-induced bradycardia in anesthetized rats. Jpn J Pharmacol 1994;65:241–8.
[83] Heesen M, Klimek M, Hoeks SE, et al. Prevention of spinal anesthesia-induced hypotension during cesarean delivery by 5-hydroxytryptamine-3 receptors antagonists: a systematic review and meta-analysis and meta-regression. Anesth Analg 2016;123:977–88.
[84] Gao L, Zheng G, Han J, et al. Effects of prophylactic ondansetron on spinal anesthesia-induced hypotension: a meta-analysis. Int J Obstet Anesth 2015;24:335–43.
[85] Karacaer F, Biricik E, Unal I, et al. Does prophylactic ondansetron reduce norepinephrine consumption in patients undergoing cesarean section with spinal anesthesia? J Anesth 2018;32:90–7.

[86] Sun LH, Ling QD, Sun WZ, et al. Lower limb wrapping prevents hypotension, but not hypothermia or shivering, after the introduction of epidural anesthesia for cesarean delivery. Anesth Analg 2004;99:241–4.
[87] Van Bogaert LJ. Prevention of post-spinal hypotension at elective cesarean section by wrapping of the lower limbs. Int J Gynaecol Obstet 1998;61:233–8.
[88] Bhagwanjee S, Rocke DA, Rout CC, et al. Prevention of hypotension following spinal anaesthesia for elective caesarean section by wrapping of the legs. Br J Anaesth 1990;65:819–22.
[89] Sood PK, Cooper PJ, Michel MZ, et al. Thromboembolic deterrent stockings fail to prevent hypotension associated with spinal anaesthesia for elective caesarean section. Int J Obstet Anesth 1996;5:172–5.
[90] Sutherland PD, Wee MY, Weston-Smith P, et al. The use of thromboembolic deterrent stockings and a sequential compression device to prevent spinal hypotension during caesarean section. Int J Obstet Anesth 2001;10:97–102.
[91] Rout CC, Rocke DA, Gouws E. Leg elevation and wrapping in the prevention of hypotension following spinal anaesthesia for elective cesarean section. Anaesthesia 1993;48:304–8.
[92] Chooi C, Cox JJ, Lumb RS, et al. Techniques for preventing hypotension during spinal anaesthesia for caesarean section. Cochrane Database Syst Rev 2017;(8):CD002251.
[93] Kuhn JC, Hauge TH, Rosseland LA, et al. Hemodynamics of phenylephrine infusion versus lower extremity compression during spinal anesthesia for cesarean delivery: a randomized, double-blind, placebo-controlled study. Anesth Analg 2016;122:1120–9.
[94] Cooper DW, Gibb SC, Meek T, et al. Effect of intravenous vasopressor on spread of spinal anesthesia and fetal acid-base equilibrium. Br J Anaesth 2007;98:649–56.
[95] Jain K, Makkar JK, Subramani Vp S, et al. A randomized trial comparing prophylactic phenylephrine and ephedrine for maintaining blood pressure during spinal anesthesia for emergency cesarean delivery in cases of acute fetal compromise. J Clin Anesth 2016;34:208–15.
[96] Clark RB, Thompson DS, Thompson CH. Prevention of spinal hypotension associated with cesarean section. Anesthesiology 1976;45:670–3.
[97] Henke VG, Bateman BT, Leffert LR. Focused review: spinal anesthesia in severe preeclampsia. Anesth Analg 2013;117:686–93.
[98] Aya AG, Mangin R, Vialles N, et al. Patients with severe preeclampsia experience less hypotension during spinal anesthesia for elective cesarean delivery than healthy parturients: a prospective cohort comparison. Anesth Analg 2003;97:867–72.
[99] Schobel HP, Fischer T, Heuszer K, et al. Preeclampsia: a state of sympathetic hyperactivity. N Engl J Med 1996;335:1480–5.
[100] Ashworth JR, Warren AY, Baker PN, et al. Loss of endothelium-dependent relaxation in myometrial resistance arteries in preeclampsia. BJOG 1997;104:1152–8.
[101] Sharwood-Smith G, Drummond GB. Hypotension in obstetric spinal anaesthesia: a lesson from pre-eclampsia. Br J Anaesth 2009;102:291–4.
[102] Lee AJ, Landau R, Mattingly JL, et al. Left lateral table tilt for elective cesarean delivery under spinal anesthesia has no effect on neonatal acid-base status. Anesthesiology 2017;127:241–9.
[103] Lee AJ, Landau R. Aortocaval compression syndrome: time to revisit certain dogmas. Anesth Analg 2017;125:1975–85.
[104] Farber MK, Bateman BT. Phenylephrine infusion: driving a wedge in our practice of left uterine displacement. Anesthesiology 2017;127:212–4.